EASY
FACIAL CUPPING
AT HOME

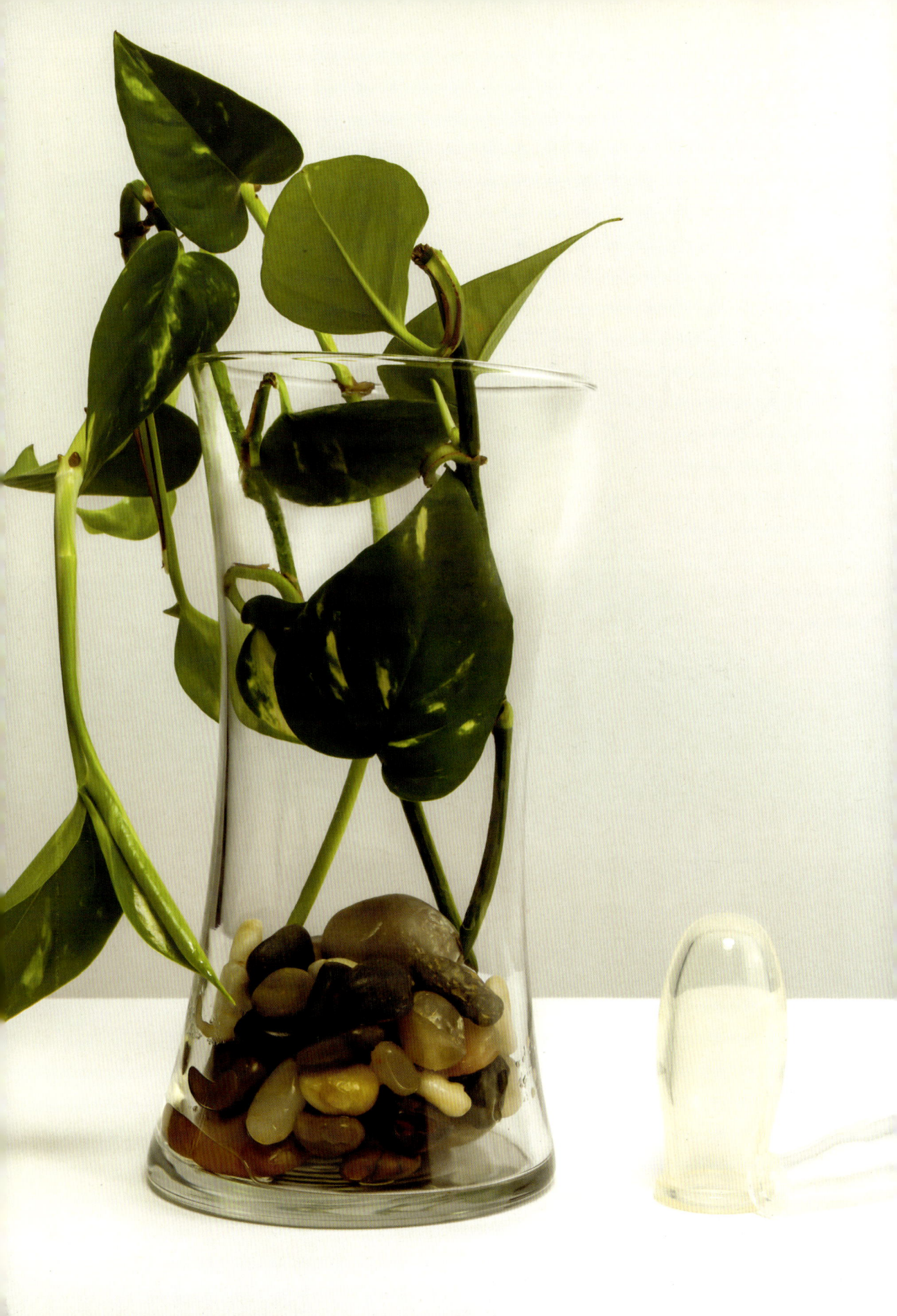

EASY
FACIAL CUPPING
AT HOME

**YOUR SIMPLE GUIDE FOR
HEALTHY, REJUVENATED SKIN**

SHANNON GILMARTIN
CMT, CMLDT, CMCTPE

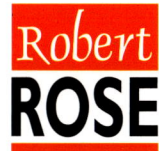

Easy Facial Cupping at Home
Text copyright © 2023 Shannon Gilmartin
Photographs copyright © 2023 Doug Arcos (except as noted below)
Cover and text design copyright © 2023 Robert Rose Inc.

No part of this publication may be reproduced, stored in a retrieval system or transmitted to any form or by any means, without the prior written consent of the publisher or a license from the Canadian Copyright Licensing Agency (Access Copyright). For an Access Copyright license, visit www.accesscopyright.ca or call toll-free: 1-800-893-5777.

For complete cataloguing information, see page 176.

Disclaimer
This book is a general guide only and should never be a substitute for the skill, knowledge and experience of a qualified medical professional dealing with the facts, circumstances and symptoms of a particular case.

The exercises, nutritional, medical and health information presented in this book is based on the research, training and professional experience of the author, and is true and complete to the best of her knowledge. However, this book is intended only as an informative guide for those wishing to know more about health, nutrition and medicine; it is not intended to replace or countermand the advice given by the reader's personal physician. Because each person and situation is unique, the author and the publisher urge the reader to check with a qualified health-care professional before using any procedure where there is a question as to its appropriateness. A physician should be consulted before beginning any exercise program. The author and the publisher are not responsible for any adverse effects or consequences resulting from the use of the information in this book. It is the responsibility of the reader to consult a physician or other qualified health-care professional regarding his or her personal care.

EDITOR: Kathleen Fraser
INDEXER: Gillian Watts
DESIGN AND PRODUCTION: PageWave Graphics Inc.
PHOTOGRAPHY: Doug Arcos

BACKGROUND TEXTURE (pages 12, 16, 18-19, 29, 32-33, 38, 41, 42-43, 50-51, 66-67, 74-75, 86, 89, 97, 104, 110, 120, 130, 140, 151, 152-153, 160, 166-167, 168, 171, 172): © Getty Images
ILLUSTRATIONS (pages 15, 21, 22, 26, 69, 80, 81, 105, 111, 121, 131, 141): © Getty Images
ADDITIONAL PHOTOGRAPHY (pages 35, 102, 158): © Getty Images

Published by Robert Rose Inc.
120 Eglinton Avenue East, Suite 800, Toronto, Ontario, Canada, M4P 1E2
Tel: (416) 322-6552 Fax: (416) 322-6936
www.robertrose.ca

Printed and bound in China

1 2 3 4 5 6 7 8 9 ESP 31 30 29 28 27 26 25 24 23

This book is dedicated to every client, student, family member and friend who has enjoyed facial cupping treatments and wished they could learn how to do it for themselves.

With great enthusiasm and gratitude for you all — enjoy!

CONTENTS

Introduction 9

CHAPTER 1
ANATOMY OF THE FACE
Anatomy of the Skin, Circulation and Muscles 20
Healthy Skin Components 28
Risk Factors and Other Elements to Consider 30

CHAPTER 2
BENEFITS OF CUPPING FOR THE FACE
Benefits for the Skin 37
Benefits for Circulation 39
Benefits for Muscles 40

CHAPTER 3
CUPPING EQUIPMENT AND PRODUCTS
Cupping Equipment 44
Cleaning and Storing Equipment 48

CHAPTER 4
USING CUPS ON THE FACE
Techniques for Facial Cupping 52
Methods of Application 61
What about Cupping Marks? (What Not to Do). 63

CHAPTER 5
SAFETY FIRST

Endangerment Sites 68
Working with Cosmetic Injections 72
Post-Surgical Considerations 73

CHAPTER 6
BEFORE YOU BEGIN

Assessing Your Skin 76
Exceptions and What-Ifs 77
Preparing for Facial Cupping 84
Know Your Limits and When to Seek Professional Help 87

CHAPTER 7
FACIAL CUPPING STEP-BY-STEP TREATMENT

Overview of Treatment Process 91
Understanding the Universal Pass 94
Step 1: The Neck and Upper Chest 105
Step 2: The Jawline 111
Step 3: The Cheeks and Upper Lip 121
Step 4: The Forehead 131
Step 5: The Eye Area 141
The Face-Cupping Map 150

CHAPTER 8
AFTER YOUR FACIAL CUPPING TREATMENT

Products to Apply 154
Make a Treatment Plan 158

The Full Potential of Therapeutic Cupping for Skin Health: My Story 161
References and Resources 169
Acknowledgments 170
Index 173

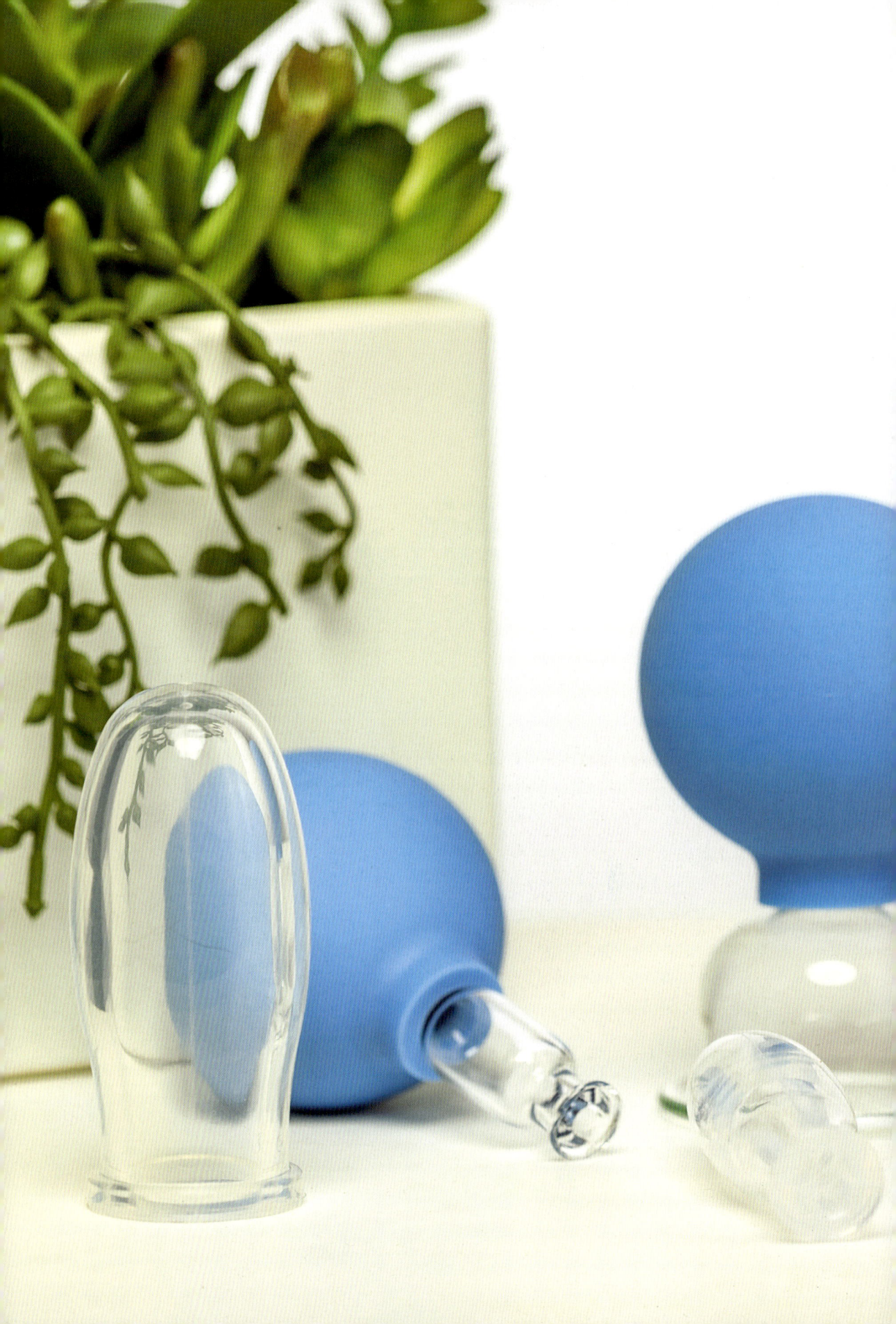

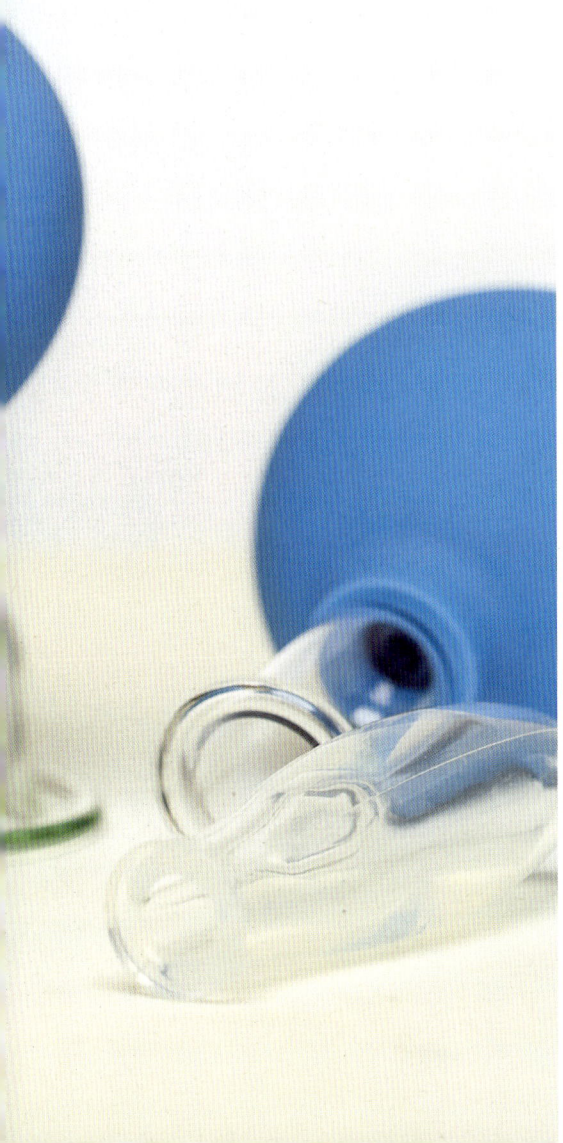

INTRODUCTION

I LOVE CUPS. With so many ways to use them, cups have become a therapeutic tool used by many people and in so many ways. And facial cupping is one of my favorite treatments. It offers natural esthetic and health benefits unlike those of any other noninvasive facial treatment option available today. And it feels good, too.

TREATING YOURSELF

I AM THRILLED to bring the knowledge I have gained through my own professional and personal experience to those who are interested in treating themselves with facial cupping.

This book will teach you safe, effective and proper methods of facial cupping that you can do on your own. Far too many people gain flawed information on the internet and, when they attempt to treat themselves, they do it incorrectly. Perhaps they leave cupping marks or bruises, or create swelling. Sadly, all of this is possible when cupping is done incorrectly. And then they give up when they don't get the promised results.

My goal with this book is to empower people to treat themselves correctly and get the awesome results I know are possible.

In this book, you'll find all the information and guidance you need. I will help you to understand the anatomy of the face, how cupping benefits every aspect of the face and what to expect for results. You will learn about the cupping equipment, how to prepare your face for the best treatment possible and what to do afterward for maximum benefit. Most importantly, you will find detailed, step-by-step, easy-to-follow instructions on how to treat your own face with facial cupping.

And I address the million-dollar question: Will I end up with cupping marks on my face? The facial cupping treatment does not mark the face 99.9 percent of the time. In this book, you will understand exactly what a cupping mark is, why they occur and how to avoid that 0.1 percent chance.

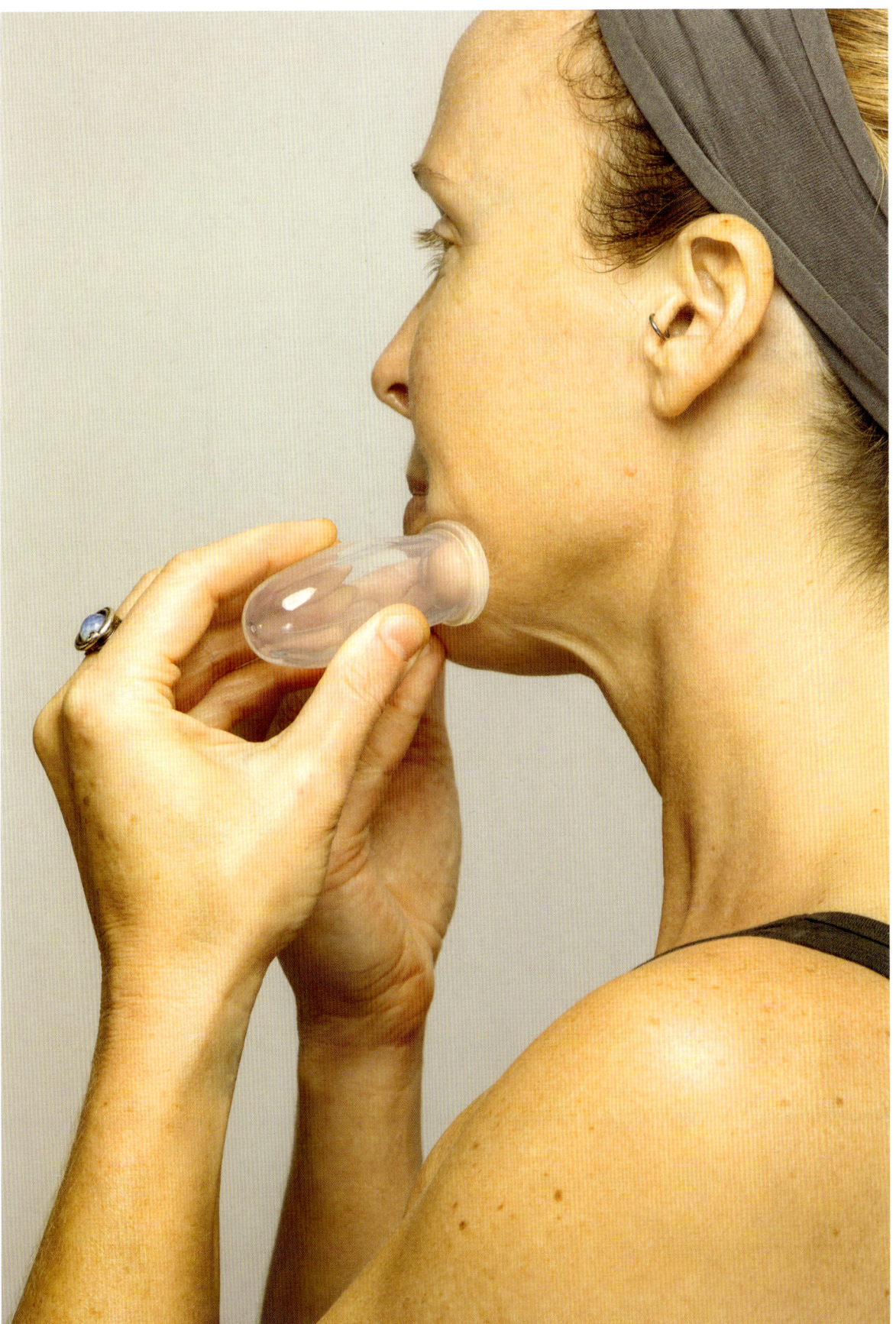

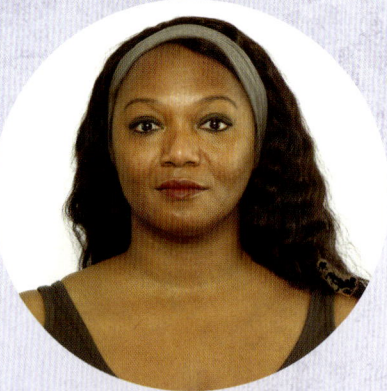
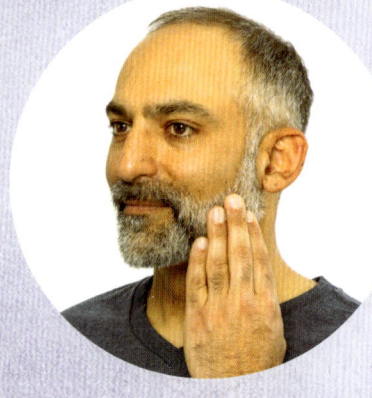
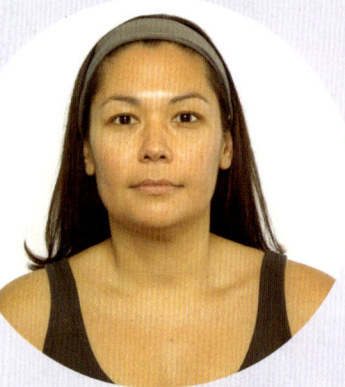

No two faces are alike.

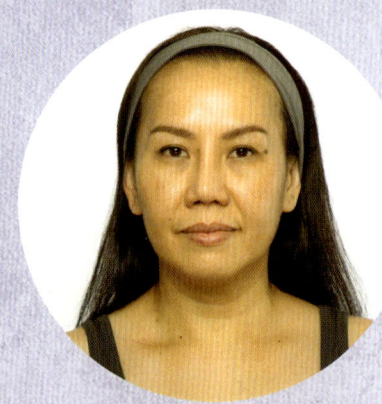
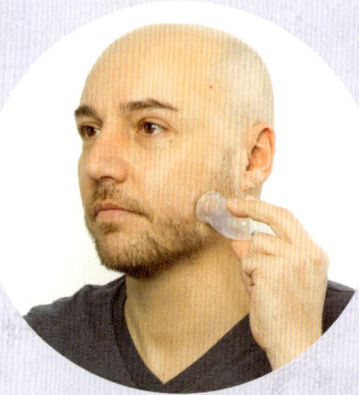
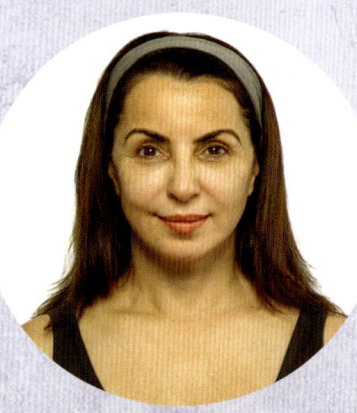

> I promise you that this is an easy treatment to do. All you have to do is invest in the process, read the directions and follow them exactly as instructed.

This book offers suggestions on how cupping can be tailored to fit your personal needs, as no two faces are alike. Do you have loose skin you want to tone up? Cupping can help. Do you have wrinkles you want to minimize without injections or surgeries? Cupping is a natural way to do that. Does your overall complexion seem as if it could use a little boost? Cupping can bring the resilience back, naturally! I often say facial cupping is like a facial, but with no products. That entices almost everyone!

Other personal needs are considered, too. For example, do you have jaw tension related to temporomandibular joint (TMJ) dysfunction? Cupping can provide relief. Do you have facial hair? I offer suggestions on how to treat the entire face, whether there is hair or not. Do you have acne? Sinus congestion? Have you had injections or other cosmetic procedures? If yes, there are suggestions on how to adjust the application so you, too, can enjoy the many benefits facial cupping has to offer.

I hope you find something useful on every page. Welcome to the wonderful world of facial cupping!

HISTORY OF CUPPING

CUPPING THERAPY has existed throughout civilized times and evidence of its usage can be found in most cultures around the world.

Body cupping has a rich history of diverse medicinal applications and has been used to treat aches and pains, diseases, digestive issues, emotional disorders and many more ailments.

Cupping for cosmetic benefits can be similarly traced back to ancient Egypt, China, many European countries and even the Americas. In those days, only wealthy families and members of high society enjoyed the benefits of cupping for maintaining a youthful appearance.

As an alternative and complimentary therapy used the world over, cupping results are difficult to measure by Western standards. As well, there are many interpretations of how to use them, and such confusion may result in inconsistent or improper usage. Cupping should never be painful. When done correctly, the results speak for themselves. People feel relief from cupping. You should find the experience of receiving cupping quite enjoyable!

While the clinical usages of body cupping have varied over the years, cupping for cosmetic rejuvenation has stayed strong in the wellness industry. During the twentieth century, when wellness spas began offering services for beauty, cupping devices began to be used along with various vibrational devices, scraping tools and other mechanical treatments. These early cupping practices were used for a variety of cosmetic purposes, including cellulite reduction and general skin treatments.

More recently, in the 1970s and 1980s, there was growing interest in cupping for facial rejuvenation. Nowadays, facial cupping is one of the most popular noninvasive services available at premier wellness facilities.

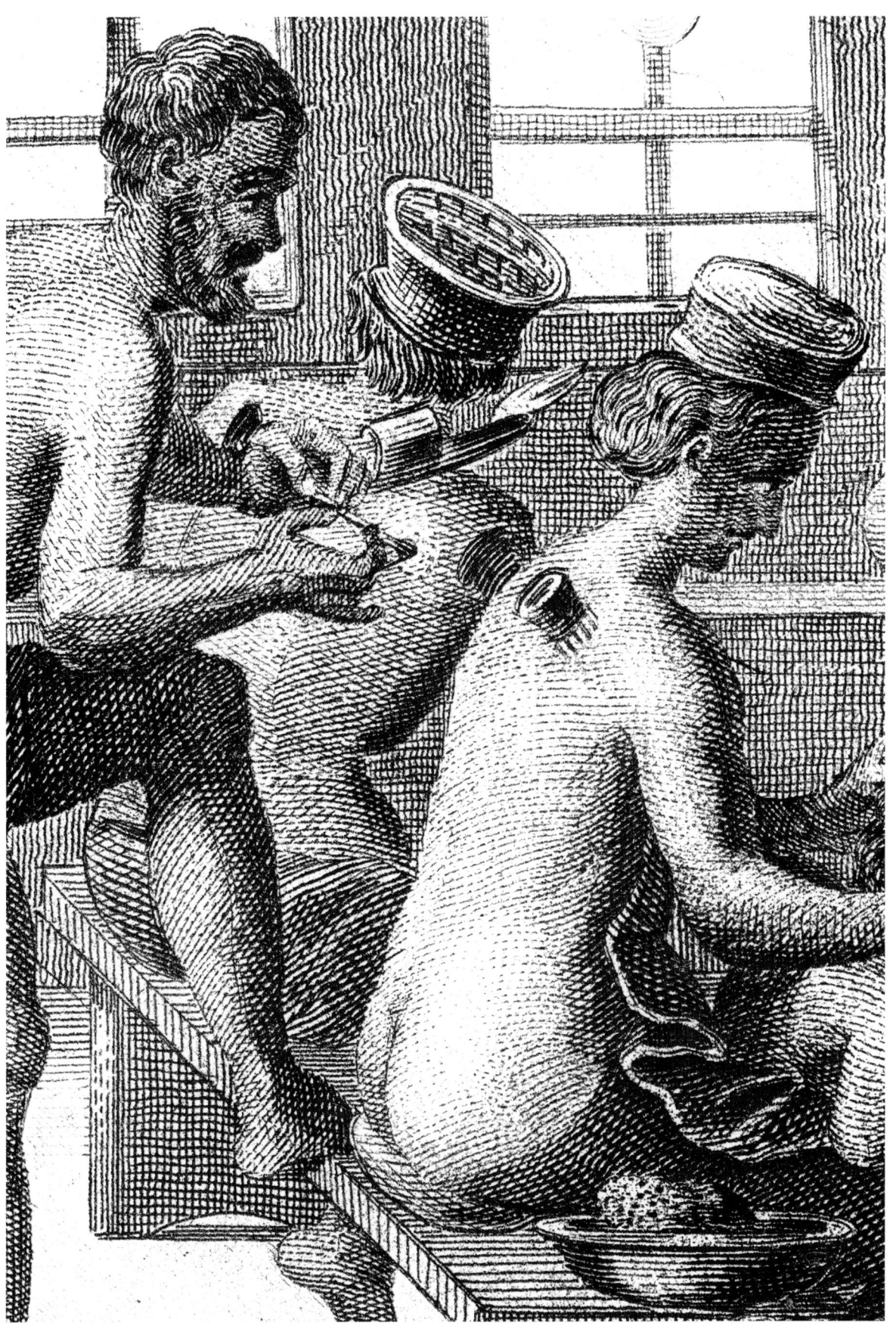

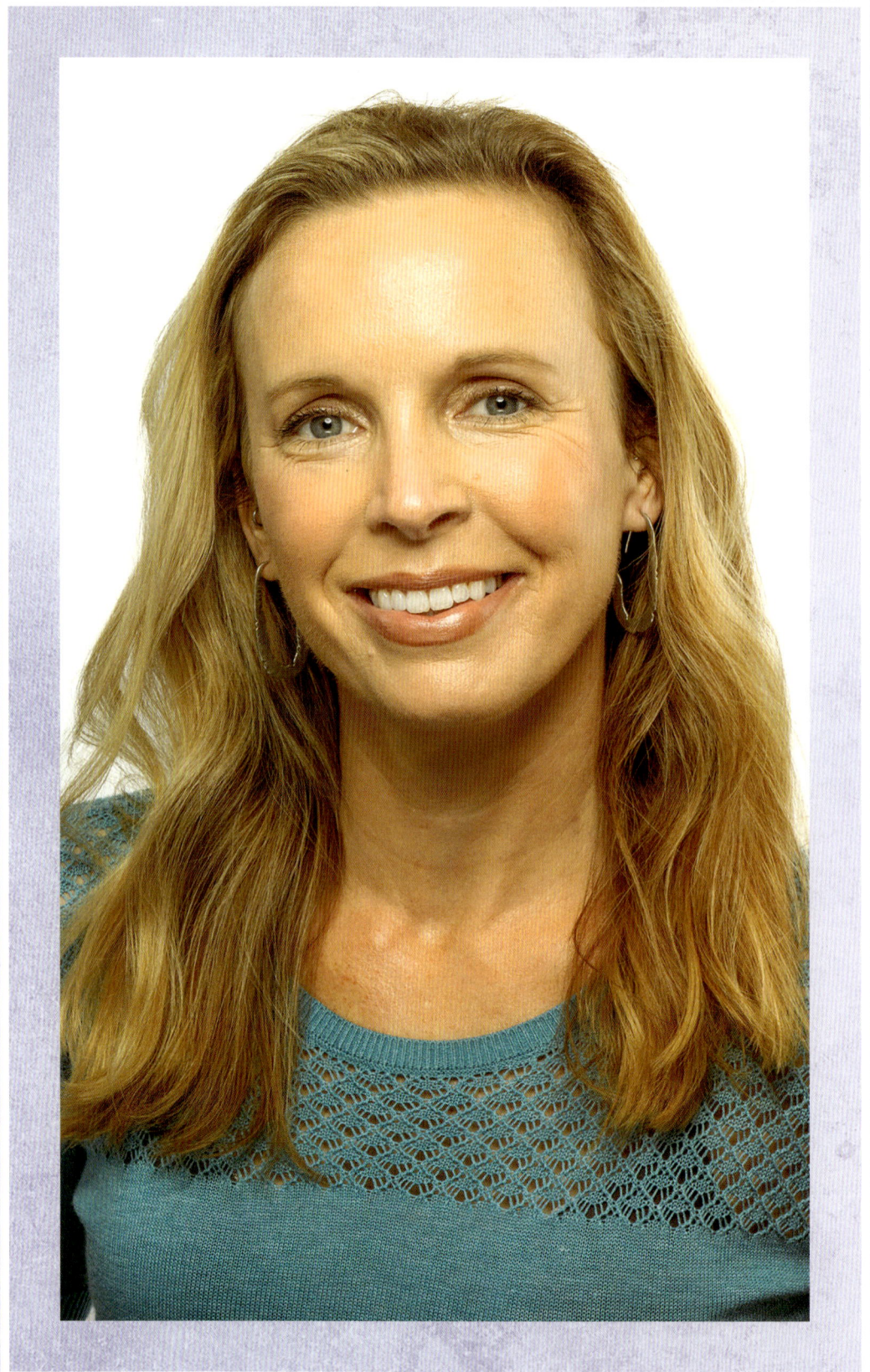

ABOUT THE AUTHOR

I STARTED my career as a professional therapeutic bodyworker in 1999. Therapeutic bodywork encompasses a number of techniques and modalities to promote health and wellness. In my case, cupping was one of the first alternative modalities I learned. It completely changed everything for me, both personally and professionally.

Every time I share my own story of facial cupping and the results, people either do not believe me, or they are shocked and even more excited to learn about this treatment for themselves. After years of chronic pain and scar tissue, cupping offered me extraordinary relief. Facial cupping was transformational for me. If you want to get excited now about the potential cupping offers, turn to page 161 at the end of this book to read more about my personal story.

In my clinical practice, cups have been the best addition to my therapeutic treatments. The way cups change soft tissue and the extraordinary results they bring my clients is unlike any other modality I have learned, ever. From relaxing treatments and deep tissue bodywork to post-surgical rehabilitative therapies and even Thai massage, cupping is the most versatile tool available to bodyworkers today. Every client who receives cupping bodywork reports enjoyable sensations and incomparable results. The feedback I receive is always positive.

As a cupping educator, I am honored to share this powerful information to people all over the world. When used correctly, cups are powerful tools that can add a whole new dimension of therapeutic benefit. And while in my classroom we have many days of course content to offer, the facial cupping part is among the most popular.

CHAPTER 1

ANATOMY OF THE FACE

Anatomy of the Skin, Circulation and Muscles
20

Healthy Skin Components
28

Risk Factors and Other Elements to Consider
30

Anatomy of the Skin, Circulation and Muscles

THE SKIN

YOUR SKIN has many layers of soft tissue that contain nerves, hair follicles and glands, and it hosts countless cellular functions that all work together to regulate and protect the body.

Your skin has three primary layers: the epidermis, the dermis and the hypodermis.

The outermost layer is the *epidermis*. It is thin, offers protection and contains many nerve endings. It is the last part of the body to receive blood flow, yet the first part we see, touch and feel.

The middle layer is the *dermis,* also known as "the true skin." It supplies the skin with oxygen and nutrients thanks to its wealth of blood and lymph vessels. The dermis also contains collagen and elastin, which are protein substances that give the skin firmness and elasticity. As natural connective tissue fibers called fibroblasts constantly work to rebuild tissues, they produce collagen and elastin; this is one of our normal cellular functions.

The deepest layer is the *hypodermis*. Also known as the subcutaneous (deep) or superficial fascia, this layer connects the skin to the underlying muscles. It is composed mostly of fatty (adipose) tissue and contains many circulatory vessels, nerves and connective tissue fibers. Because this layer decreases with age, maintaining its wellness throughout our lives is vital to ensuring the health of the other, more superficial layers of skin.

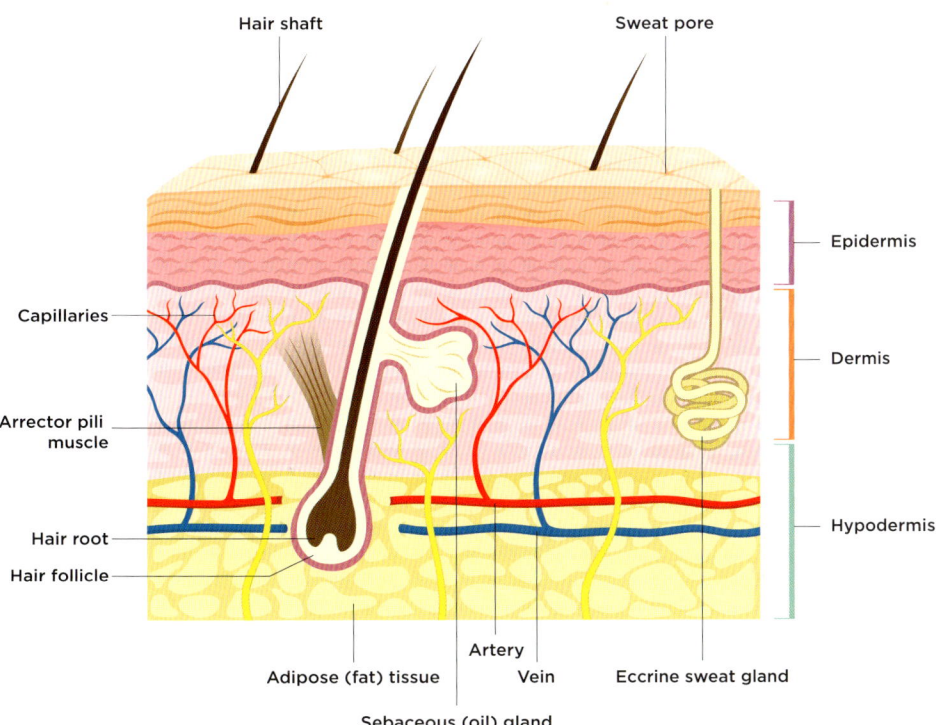

The skin is the largest organ of the body and yet it is one of the last to receive blood flow. Maintaining a healthy appearance requires support not only from the outside but, more importantly, from the inside body systems that nourish the skin. Although the composition of our skin is generally the same among all humans, individually our skin is what identifies us and gives each of us our own unique appearance.

CIRCULATION

THE SKIN IS NOURISHED, maintained and detoxified by our *circulatory system*, which connects and circulates through the many layers of our bodies. A harmonious flow of blood and nutrient distribution, waste collection and filtration occurs within this body system. For ease of understanding, we divide this complex system into two parts: the cardiovascular and lymphovascular systems.

The *cardiovascular system* is one part of the circulatory system that involves blood movement. Its many functions include the distribution of respiratory gases (oxygen and carbon dioxide), nutrients, antibodies and hormones. It also supports immune system functions by producing various disease-fighting cells, including red and white blood cells, protects the body from excessive loss of bodily fluids from traumas by clotting and helps regulate body temperature through perspiration.

BLOOD VESSELS OF THE FACE

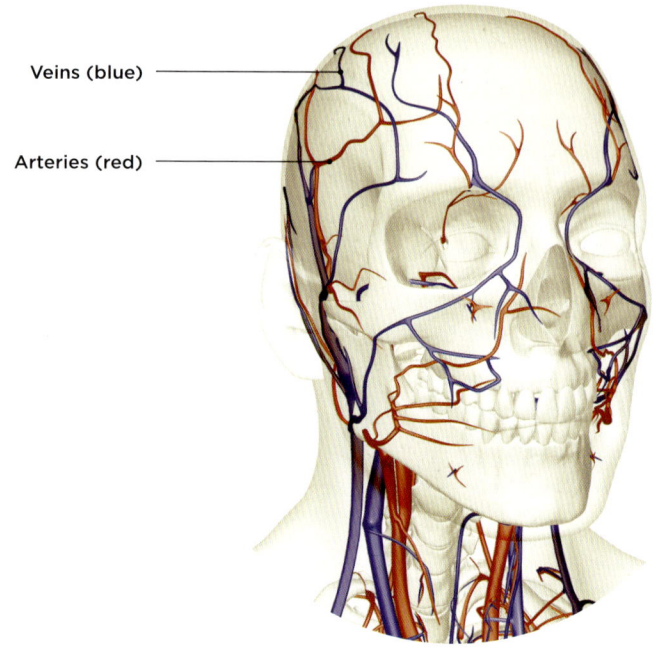

Blood vessels are tubes that carry blood both into and out of the heart, weaving throughout our bodies for thousands of miles. Blood distributes oxygen and vital nutrients — including those responsible for assisting with the production of collagen and elastin — into all parts of the body while simultaneously removing waste products from these same locations.

Blood moves with various muscle contractions; when it leaves the heart, blood is pumped out through arteries, which decrease in size, eventually reaching the smallest segments, which are called capillaries. These capillaries are responsible for distributing nutrient- and oxygen-rich blood to thousands of end points throughout our body, including the skin and muscle tissues. Blood flow at this capillary level is called *microcirculation*. At these end points, capillaries meet venules (the smallest segments of veins) that collect nutrient-deficient blood and carbon dioxide waste. The venules progressively grow into larger veins — some identifiable under the skin's surface — ultimately ending at the heart where the cycle begins again.

Amid all this blood movement, blood also enters and exits the lungs, for carbon dioxide removal and oxygen replenishment. This cycle is constant and is vital to all of life's functions, especially overall health and wellness.

The other part of our cardiovascular system is the *lymphovascular or lymphatic system*, which controls lymph circulation. The lymphatic system exists alongside the cardiovascular system but has a circuitry all its own, involving many types of vessels, nodes and organs including the spleen, thymus gland and tonsils. The lymphatic system is responsible for filtration of lymph fluids and harmful pathogenic substances, delivers fats and vitamins from the digestive system into circulation and offers major defensive support to the immune system.

Lymph fluids consist of water, various cells and waste materials, including protein particles (not reabsorbed by capillaries) and any foreign or pathogenic substances such as environmental toxic exposures, bacteria and cancer cells.

The lymphatic system follows its own complex drainage route, clearing sections of the body in a logical, holistic manner. Most of its collection begins at skin level with lymph capillaries, which attach to the underside of the skin and exist in the outermost layers of soft tissue. After collection, lymph fluids are moved along an intricate route of filtration, fluid recirculation and bodily waste removal. Lymph drainage ends at the upper chest, where these filtered fluids are returned to your blood circulation through your veins. Optimal lymph drainage is crucial for general wellness.

The movement of lymph can become challenged for many reasons. Lymph generally moves by three mechanisms: breathing, muscle contraction and manual therapy. While we can do breathing and muscle contractions on our own, manual therapies are very useful to promote lymph drainage.

For this reason, there is a specific skillset some bodywork and skincare professionals are trained in known as manual lymph drainage. Because the lymph capillaries are located just underneath the skin, therapists can easily influence lymph drainage by using light pressure manually applied to the skin. Following the correct drainage routes is crucial, as the direction of lymph drainage is easily influenced at this superficial level. Therefore, light pressure and specific directions for application are key to promoting optimal lymph drainage.

Lymph drainage treatments are a major component of most skincare professional services, and optimal lymph drainage is one of the best natural ways to improve and maintain healthy, beautiful skin.

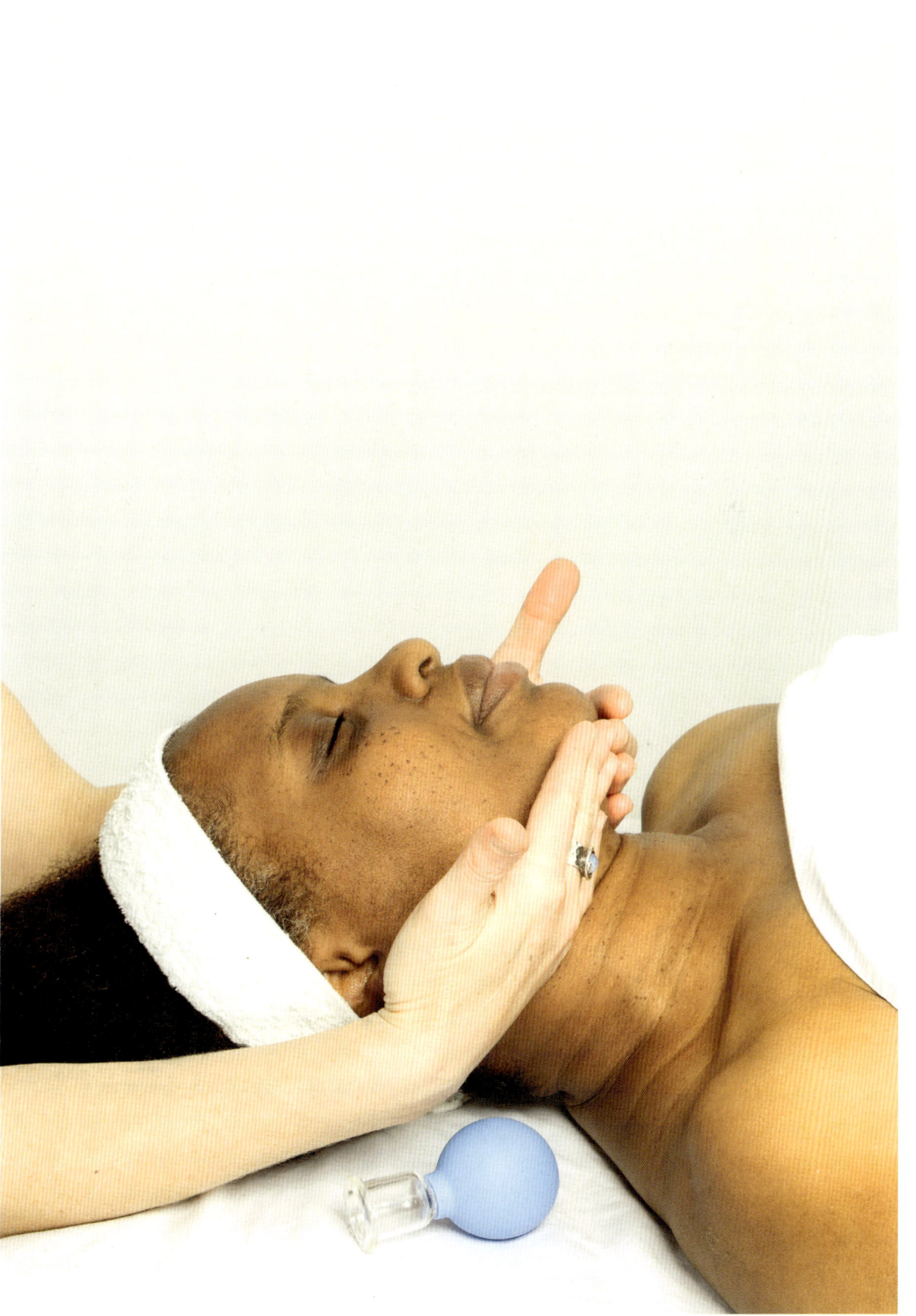

MUSCLES

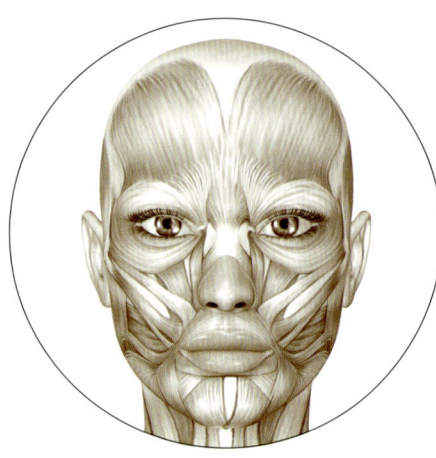 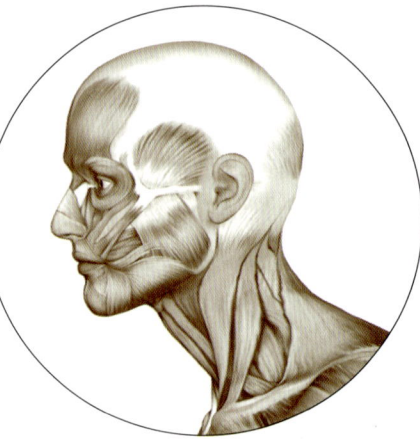

OUR MUSCLES are responsible for many things; they help us maintain posture and stability, support overall circulation of blood and lymph, control smooth muscle contractions in our visceral organs (such as the contractions that allow food in the digestive tract to move through the body), support body temperature regulation and move our bodies.

There are three types of muscles — skeletal, smooth and cardiac — and our skeletal muscles are the ones responsible for movement, including facial expressions. Just under your skin you will find connections to the skeletal muscles. Of approximately 650 muscles in the body, our faces contain about 20. Muscles contract and relax. They require hydration to maintain suppleness and optimal function.

Muscles not only create the many facial expressions we show, but their actions help move blood and lymph along their routes. Muscular *adhesions*, or restrictions, can occur for many reasons; in the face, this can contribute to wrinkles as well as general tension and discomfort.

Wrinkles are formed from repetitive muscular contractions, like those that occur when you make the same facial expressions repeatedly. These restrictions are adhesions that set into the skin, muscles and *fascia*, which attach and pull on the underside of the skin, thus creating the creases and indentions on the skin's surface known as wrinkles.

Muscular restrictions can also contribute to aches and discomforts anywhere in the body, even in the face. The most common sites of facial tension are in the jaw (TMJ dysfunction), forehead and neck regions.

ANATOMY FYI

Adhesions are defined as any two or more anatomical structures stuck together that shouldn't naturally be. These "stuck" areas are generally formed from injuries, inflammation or repetitive actions. Adhesions (also described as restrictions) inhibit circulation, lymph drainage and muscle relaxation. This applies to wrinkles that form between skin, muscle and fascia, and how cellulite dimples form over other parts of the body.

Fascia is connective tissue that exists in every part of the body. Fascia is involved with every tissue structure (including skin, circulatory vessels, muscles, organs and bones), envelops every part of our anatomy and holds our bodies together.

Healthy Skin Components

WITH GOOD CIRCULATION of blood and lymph, healthy tissue functions thrive, muscles perform at their best and our skin remains healthy. Healthy skin requires not only optimal circulation and muscle tone, but also good hydration and nutrition and environmental support (such as sunscreen and good cleaning habits) for it to look and feel its best.

The human body is about 70 percent water, which means a good volume of daily water intake is vital to maintain optimal bodily functions. Water keeps blood flowing, lymph moving, muscles functioning and skin healthy. Make sure you drink enough water every day.

A well-balanced, healthy diet also helps to maintain skin health. There are countless resources including books, articles and nutritional experts that offer information on what a healthy diet is for you. They can advise you on the best foods and supplements for healthy skin. Do your best to feed your skin from the inside out.

Also, using quality skincare products is important for supporting healthy skin from the outside. Simple skincare regimens that include washing, moisturizing and sunscreen are ideal. Consult a skincare professional for useful insight into your personal needs.

> **WATER INTAKE FYI**
> While measurements may vary, there are a few general suggestions on how much water you should drink. One recommendation is to drink approximately nine glasses of water daily. Another way to calculate your ideal water intake is to divide your body weight in half and drink that amount of water in ounces. For example, if you weigh 140 pounds, 70 ounces of water daily is recommended.

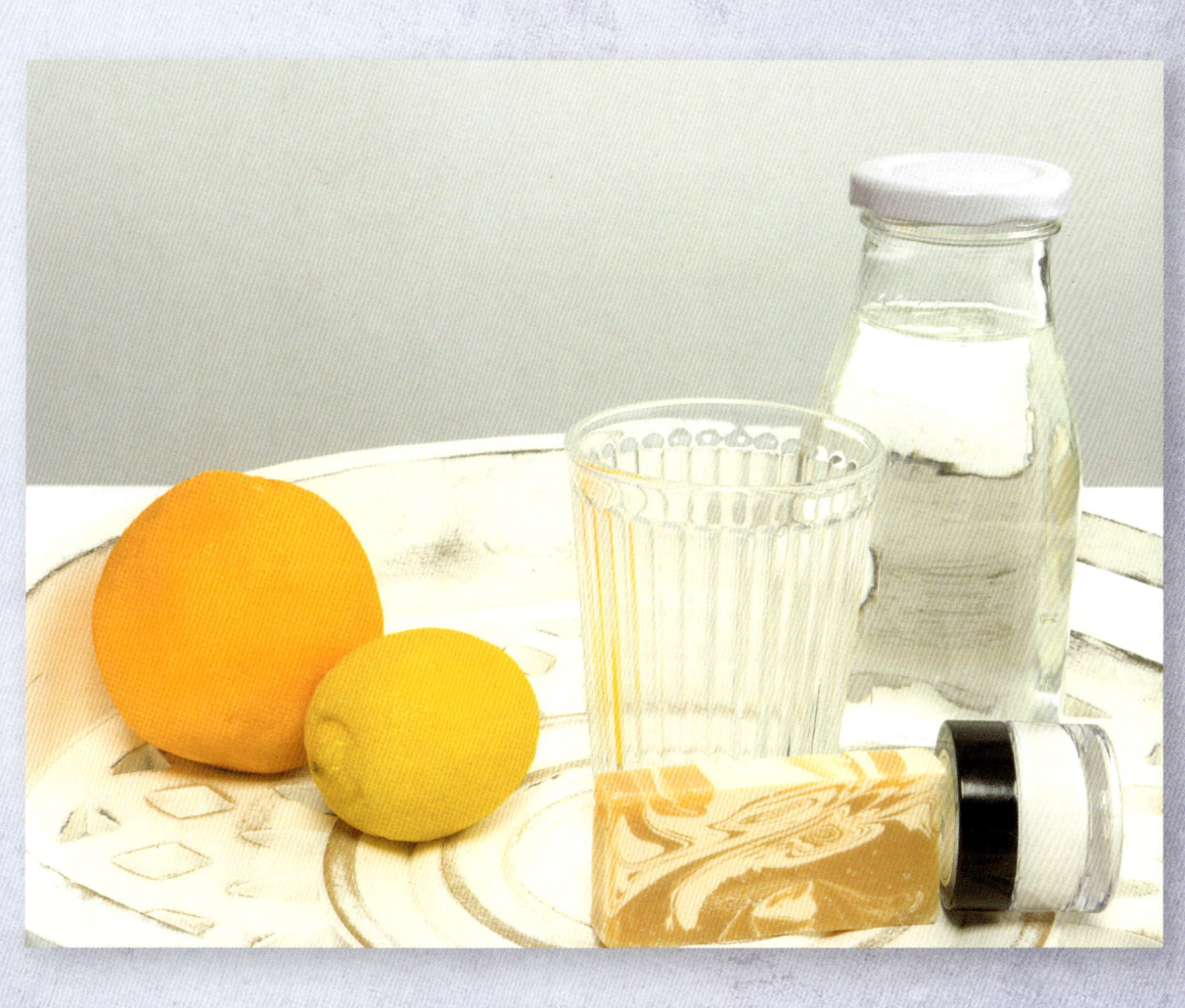

Risk Factors and Other Elements to Consider

MANY RISK FACTORS and other elements can affect the overall appearance of our skin. While there are some things we cannot control, there are others we can control; being proactive is your best option to retain a healthy complexion and overall appearance.

Dehydration and poor nutrition are major contributing factors to poor skin health. Since the skin is the last to receive blood flow, it is also the first to show signs of dehydration. Additionally, diets that are less than healthy — such as those that include highly processed foods — do not provide all the nutrients our bodies need to operate at their best. Dehydrated, malnourished skin and underlying muscles not only show a dull appearance but can also form adhesions that contribute to visible distortions on the surface of the skin, such as wrinkles and sagging skin.

Environmental factors such as air pollution and sun exposure are just two elements that cause skin damage. As we age, collagen and elastin naturally weaken in the skin, but when exposed to ultraviolet (UV) rays from the sun, this process is accelerated, potentially causing visible skin damage. Additionally, exposure to air pollution and environmental changes can irritate the skin's surface, leading to potential underlying issues if the surface is not cleaned and maintained on a regular basis.

Over time our circulatory system slows down, which contributes to inadequate blood and lymph flow and decreases the production of cells that contribute to our skin's health, including collagen and proteins. Part of a slower circulatory system includes poor lymphatic drainage, which is another major contributing factor to unhealthy skin.

Aging is inevitable and our body responds accordingly.

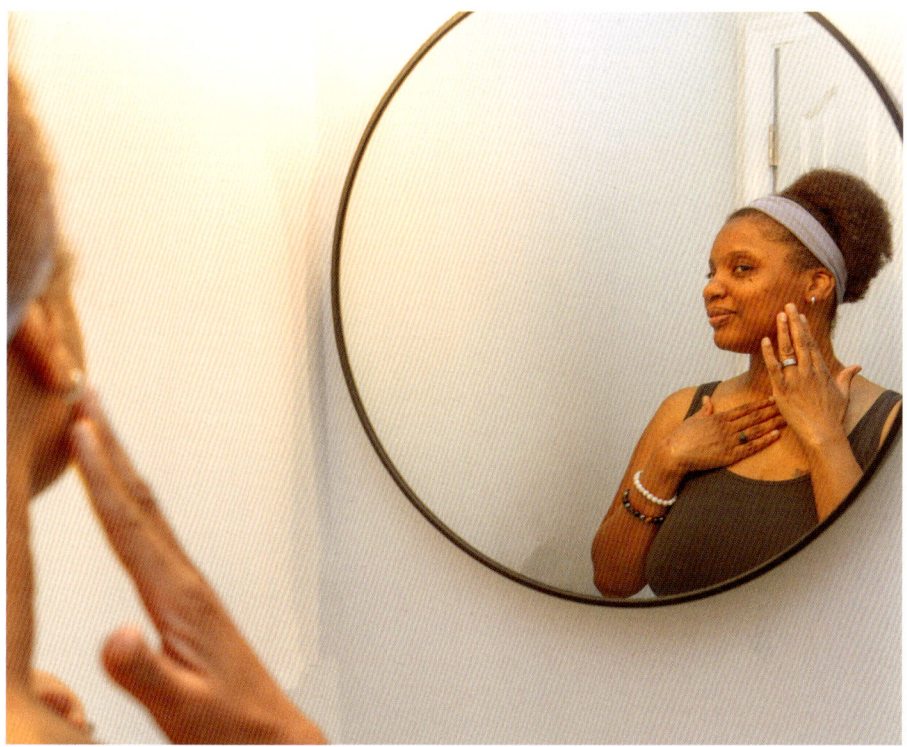

When lymph drainage is inhibited, an excess of lymph fluid can remain in the tissues, which can create not only stagnation of these lymph waste materials but also inhibits healthy blood circulation since there is no cellular space to move blood through. This creates systemic backup, which ultimately leaves skin and muscles malnourished and unhealthy.

CHAPTER 2

BENEFITS OF CUPPING FOR THE FACE

Benefits for the Skin
37

Benefits for Circulation
39

Benefits for Muscles
40

BEFORE

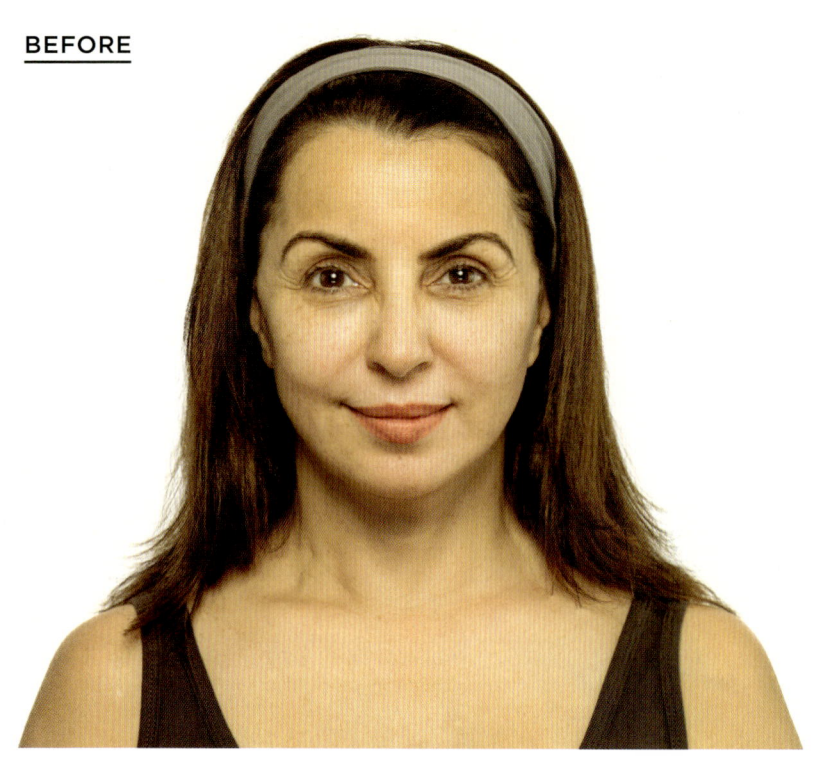

AFTER ONE TREATMENT

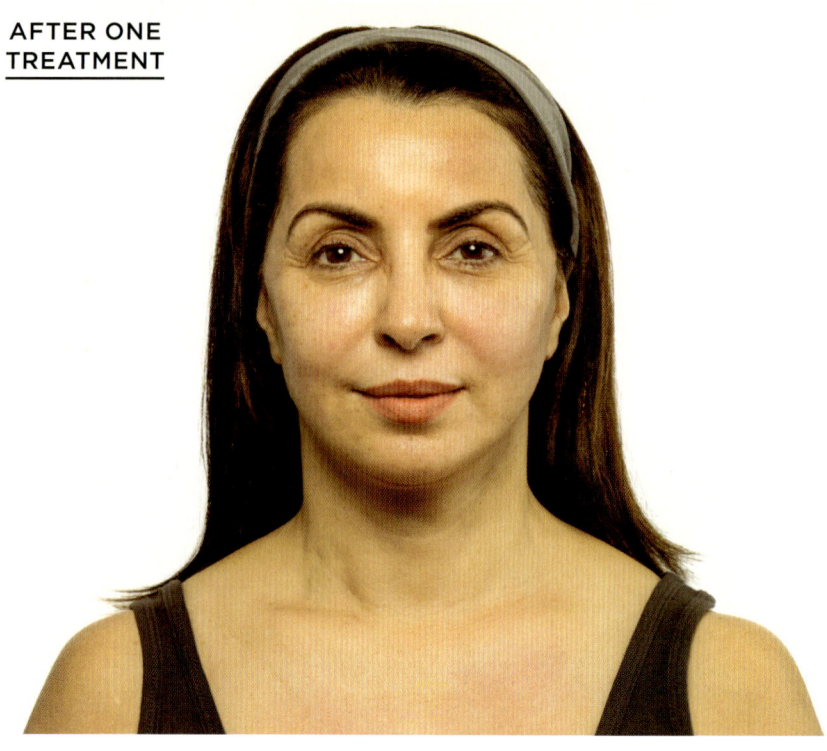

AMONG THE MANY skincare treatments and cosmetic procedures to choose from, cupping is one of the most popular, noninvasive modalities. It provides a world of benefits to the face as well as great therapeutic benefits to the rest of the body — and it feels amazing!

Cupping plumps facial tissues, boosts collagen production, improves lymph drainage and relaxes tight muscles without much effort and with no tissue damage.

To make it all possible, we rely on the three primary *physiological responses* to cups on the body: negative pressure, vasodilation and enhanced fluid exchange.

> **PHYSIOLOGY**
> The term *physiology* refers to how a body operates, its normal bodily functions. *Physiological response* refers to the way a body naturally responses to something, such as an external stimulus.

NEGATIVE PRESSURE means that cupping takes effect with a lifting of the tissues. It is different from hands-on treatments such as massage that use positive pressure, that is, pressing into the skin, to evoke a physiological response. Cups offer similar responses but with a lifting and pulling reaction anywhere they're applied. Think of this negative pressure as plumping the skin, pulling in nutrient-rich blood flow and releasing indentations where tissues are compressed.

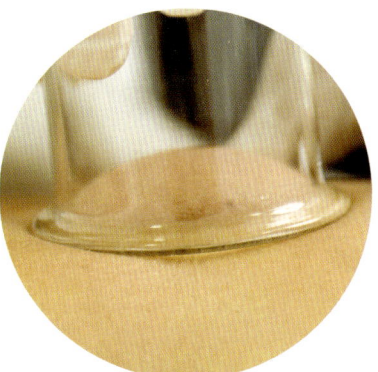

VASODILATION is a physiological response to this applied negative pressure, which allows for vessels — such as blood and lymph capillaries — to expand, thereby improving their functions. This dilating response even affects the pores in our skin, aiding in cleansing the skin and helping it to better absorb skincare products. Again, while hands-on treatments increase vascular dilation to encourage circulation of blood and lymph, cupping does this with negative pressure, which allows for the next response — enhanced fluid exchange — to be so powerful.

ENHANCED FLUID EXCHANGE occurs after the vessels are dilated; this response improves microcirculation and lymph drainage. The term *microcirculation* refers to this superficial, capillary-level process that is most involved with blood circulation at the skin level.

When you consider the combined effect of these three actions, the many benefits of cupping can be easier to understand. Cups affect the surface layers with negative pressure, so wrinkles and tension diminish easily and without discomfort. Cups improve all circulatory processes in the skin, which is one of the first goals of cosmetic improvement.

> While the effects of these three actions on the skin's surface offer many therapeutic benefits to the entire body, the skin, circulation and muscles in your face especially receive a multitude of benefits from these wonderful tools.

Benefits for the Skin
HOW CUPPING IMPROVES OVERALL APPEARANCE, TONE AND TEXTURE

SINCE CUPPING HELPS to boost microcirculation, the overall health of facial tissues is improved from the inside out.

First and foremost, improved blood flow into the deeper hypodermis allows for an increase of nutrient distribution to the dermis, which ultimately improves the appearance of the epidermis.

Also, when blood distribution improves, so do our cellular functions. This enhances cellular repair, allowing the ever-working fibroblasts to produce more collagen and elastin, inevitably resulting in a generally healthy, soft, supple and toned appearance.

While so many facial treatments and cosmetic procedures offer to boost levels of collagen and elastin — some by way of injections — cupping can offer natural, subtle and effective increases of these organic materials.

Part of what makes skin healthier is the improved circulation, which is easily visible at the skin level when a healthy glow appears after facial cupping. Furthermore, improved lymph drainage allows skin tone to improve and loose skin to tighten and makes facial rejuvenation easily accessible without any invasive procedures.

Additionally, since cupping encourages vasodilation, our pores are more open after cupping treatments. This is beneficial to the skin both as a means of cleaning the pores and also for increased product absorption. In *Chapter 8: After Your Facial Cupping Treatment*, we will discuss after-care recommendations and how applying your favorite skincare products *after* cupping is best. But no matter which topical products are applied, healthy skin always starts from the inside.

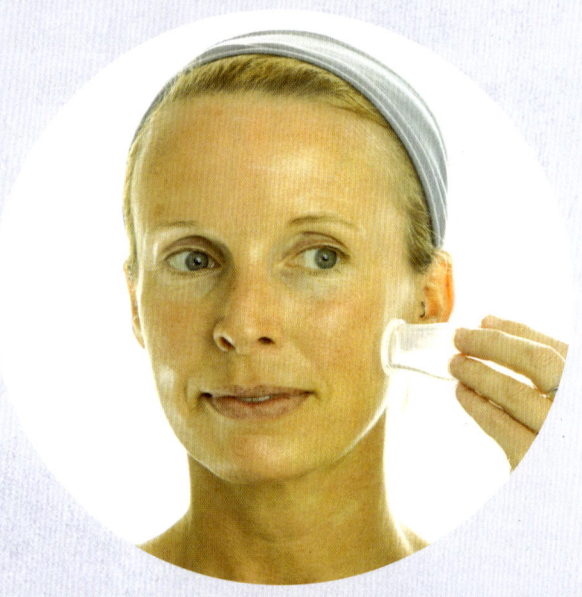

When people ask how facial cupping helps with cosmetic appearance, I say it is like a facial with no products.

Benefits for Circulation
HOW CUPS STIMULATE OVERALL CIRCULATION FOR IMPROVED ESTHETIC APPEARANCE

ONE OF THE greatest benefits of cupping is how it increases microcirculation. Countless cosmetic treatments and procedures strive to improve these systematic processes, but since cups naturally stimulate microcirculation, cupping is one of its easiest ways to achieve these benefits.

First and foremost, stimulating blood flow is what makes the skin look and feel so healthy. Improved blood flow provides an increase in nutrient and oxygen distribution to the surface layers of soft tissue. This boosts cellular functions and collagen production and results in an overall softer, healthier complexion.

At the same time, the benefits of cupping for the lymphatic system are also impressive. Good lymph drainage plays a major role in maintaining healthy skin. For this reason, the facial cupping treatment described in this book follows the natural drainage pathways of the face and head, which drain into the upper chest. Whenever you use positive pressure, there is the potential for compressing the soft tissues. But with the light, negative suction pressure of facial cupping, the influence over these superficial drainage pathways across the face is quite powerful yet has no harmful effects.

Skincare specialists agree that improved lymph drainage is just as important as improved blood flow, so the ability to increase both blood and lymph flow with negative pressure is an effective, natural way to improve your overall appearance.

Benefits for Muscles
HOW CUPPING AFFECTS MUSCLES TO REDUCE WRINKLES

CUPPING IS such a great way to address wrinkles and muscle tension! While cups may be best known for relieving muscle tension in other areas of the body, the muscles of the face receive just as much benefit from this subtle yet powerful treatment.

Think of how wrinkles are formed. They are "kinks" in the muscles. As the adhesions set into muscles (which attach to the underside of the skin), the skin's surface gets pulled inward, thus creating wrinkles. Since one of the primary responses to cupping is negative pressure, the skin and muscles are lifted when the cup is applied, which creates an outward stretch, allowing for some impressive relief of the wrinkles.

To add more benefit, the improved circulation through muscle tissue supports blood and lymph movement in the area, which in turn relaxes often-tight facial muscles with negative pressure. Instead of pressing into muscle to massage it, cups lift muscle and create relaxation with more space!

Additionally, this facial cupping treatment offers relief to other muscle tension in the face and head. Whether the discomforts are related to jaw tension, headaches or some neck pains, the entire facial cupping treatment offers great relief from many common restricted or tight areas across the face and neck.

One of my clients told me that it felt like the cupping treatment drained the stress from her face — how great does that sound?

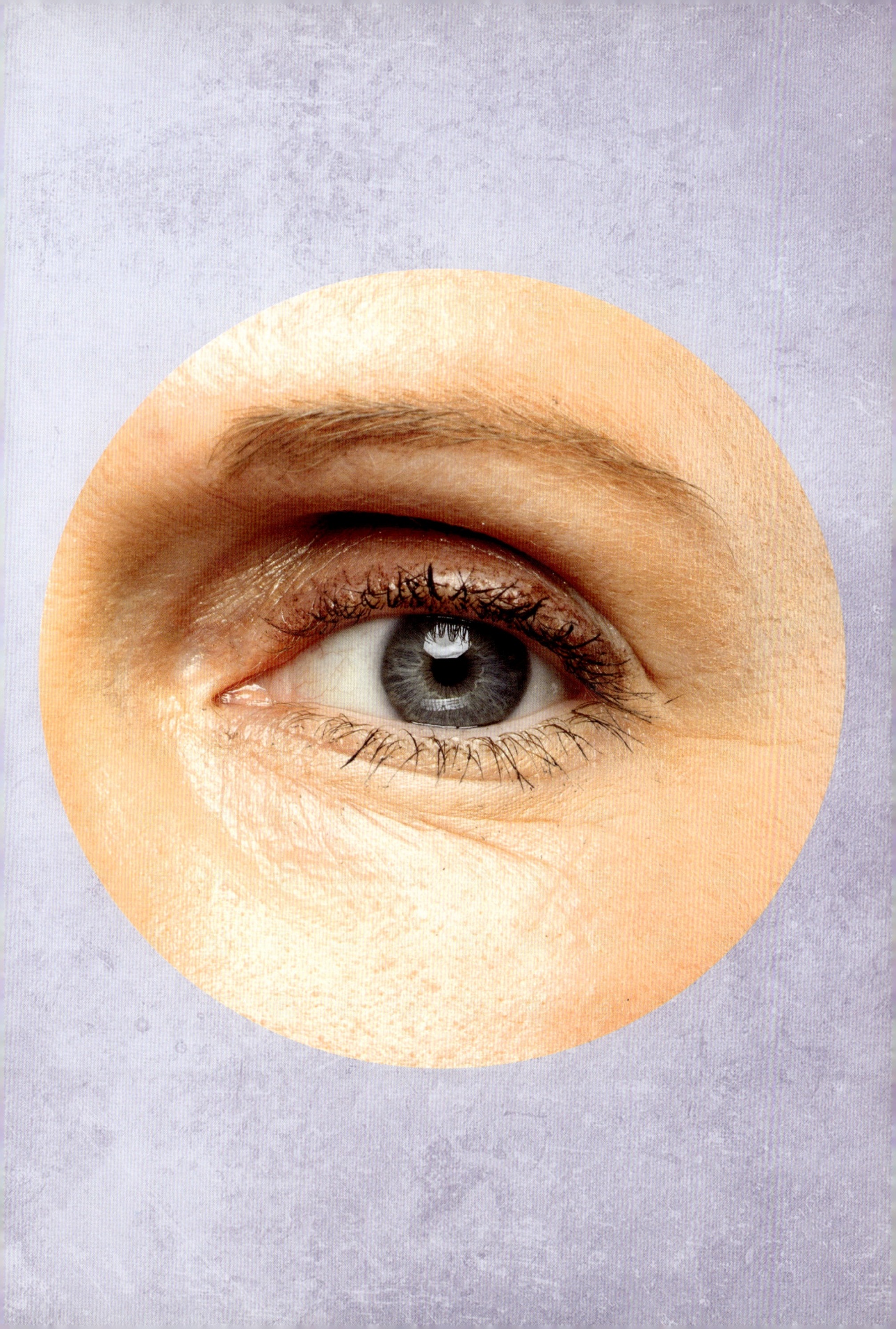

CHAPTER 3

CUPPING EQUIPMENT AND PRODUCTS

Cupping Equipment
44

Cleaning and Storing Equipment
48

Cupping Equipment

THERE ARE all sorts of cupping sets made of various materials on the market today, but for facial cupping, there are only a few options to consider.

As with any product, it's important to work with the kinds of cups that best suit your personal needs, preferences and budget. While the most common face cups are made of either glass or silicone, silicone cups are the most recommended for personal care. Not only are they the easiest to apply, but the silicone cups won't break like glass will if you accidentally drop them.

> Silicone cups are most recommended for personal care.

Additionally, silicone cups generally have less suction pressure than other cupping sets. While suction pressure with silicone cups can still be strong, the strongest suction pressure you can get from squeezing them is generally safe and easy for everyone.

Glass cupping sets or expensive cupping machines should be left to the professionals, as advanced training is necessary for using this more complicated equipment. For the purposes of this book, we will focus on using silicone face cups.

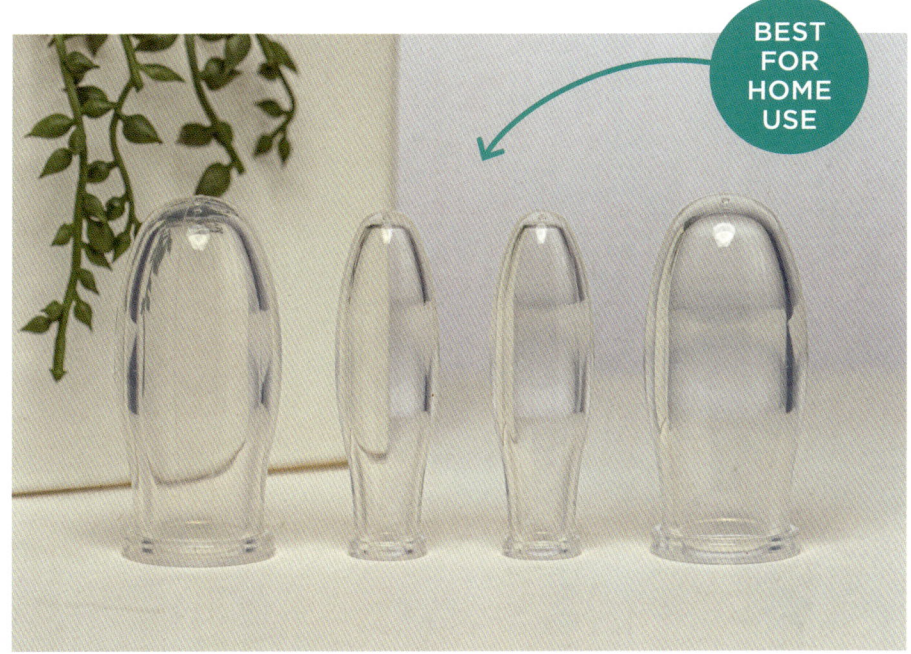

Silicone cups like these (above) are most recommended for self-care.

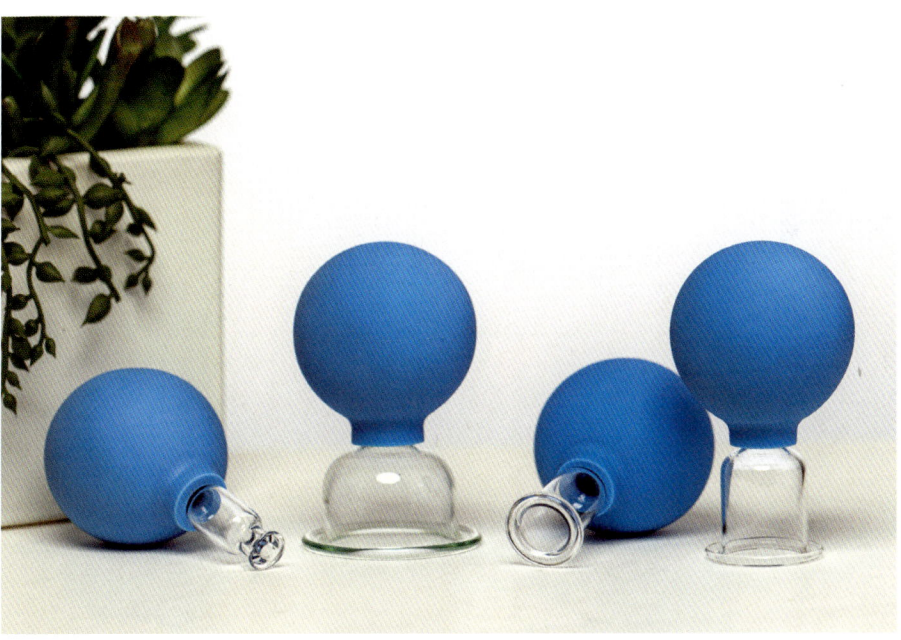

Glass cups and other costly cupping equipment are best used by trained professionals.

Most silicone face cups are easy to use. You simply squeeze them to create suction, attach them to the skin's surface and release the squeeze while maintaining your grip of the cup to engage suction on the face; then you squeeze them to detach them from the skin. I always recommend trying this method of application on your arm or upper chest before attempting it on your delicate face tissues. (We will discuss suction pressures more in the next chapter.)

The main thing you need to know is that silicone cups are easy to use and therefore best for self-care.

FAQ I'VE BEEN LOOKING AT SILICONE CUPS, AND THERE ARE A LOT OF DIFFERENT SETS AVAILABLE. WILL I GET BETTER RESULTS WITH ANY PARTICULAR SET?
No! The results will always depend on how you use the cups, not what kind of cups you have.

LUBRICANT

WHEN USING CUPS, there must be some lubricating medium between the cup and the skin's surface to create a seal. For that reason, we apply products to do just that. Additionally, cups require a slippery lubricant to move across the skin, which makes oil the best option for any cupping treatment. Some people may not like to use oil on their skin, but using a quality oil is key to this treatment.

Oil not only provides the necessary lubrication for any cupping, but it also has hydrating, nourishing and protective properties for your skin — if you choose the right one.

Many oils in your pantry are great for your skin. I say that if I can eat it, it can go on my skin! Some of the best options are olive oil or avocado oil, but any light, natural oil will do. Other oils to consider are jojoba oil, fractionated coconut oil, fragrance-free sesame oil or almond oil.

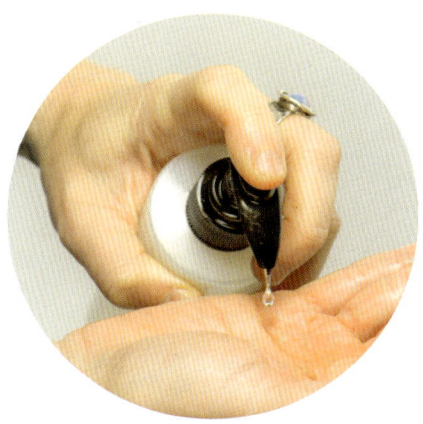

HOW MUCH OIL IS REQUIRED?

You will need enough oil to create a thin layer on the surface of the skin, but not so much that the oil is dripping off. Approximately a coin-sized amount of oil should cover your face sufficiently. If your skin is overly dry you may require more; if your skin is well hydrated you may not need as much.

No matter your previous experience, facial cupping requires more oil than you may think, especially when attempting to slide the cup on the skin. If there is too little lubricant, the cups will not move easily. That can not only be painful but it could also potentially produce cupping marks or even damage the skin. Apply plenty of oil at first, then wipe it from your hands with a cloth or towel before you pick up the cup.

DO NOT USE:

- **THICK OILS (FOR EXAMPLE, GRAPESEED OIL).** Thick oils are difficult to properly clean from the cup's surface and they don't have enough "slip" to move cups easily.

- **SOLID COCONUT OIL.** While it is great for your skin care and absorption, it can congeal on the cup and be difficult to remove. Use fractionated coconut oil instead.

- **BABY OIL OR MINERAL OIL.** Neither of these types of oils are recommended for use on facial skin.

Cleaning and Storing Equipment

CLEANING

WASHING YOUR CUPS with antibacterial soap is the minimum requirement to ensure they have a long, clean life.

While a simple washing is enough for general self-care purposes, if you prefer to also disinfect your cups there are several products on the market that will work. (See the *References and Resources* section on page 169 for more information.) For example, if you accidentally encounter any blood or sebum — if a pimple pops — then it is important to disinfect your cups after washing.

For personal usage, rubbing alcohol will work; you may either spray it over the clean cup after it has been washed or use an alcohol wipe. After you have washed your cups, a simple air drying will be enough, or you may towel dry them if you prefer.

STORING

BE SURE NOT TO store the cups with any moisture in or on the cup, as mold may grow if the cups are left to retain moisture, especially when kept in dark spaces like your cabinet or closet.

> **PRODUCT SPECIFICATIONS**
> Beyond the general usage and cleaning instructions detailed in this chapter, be sure to check package information of any set of cups for their proper care.

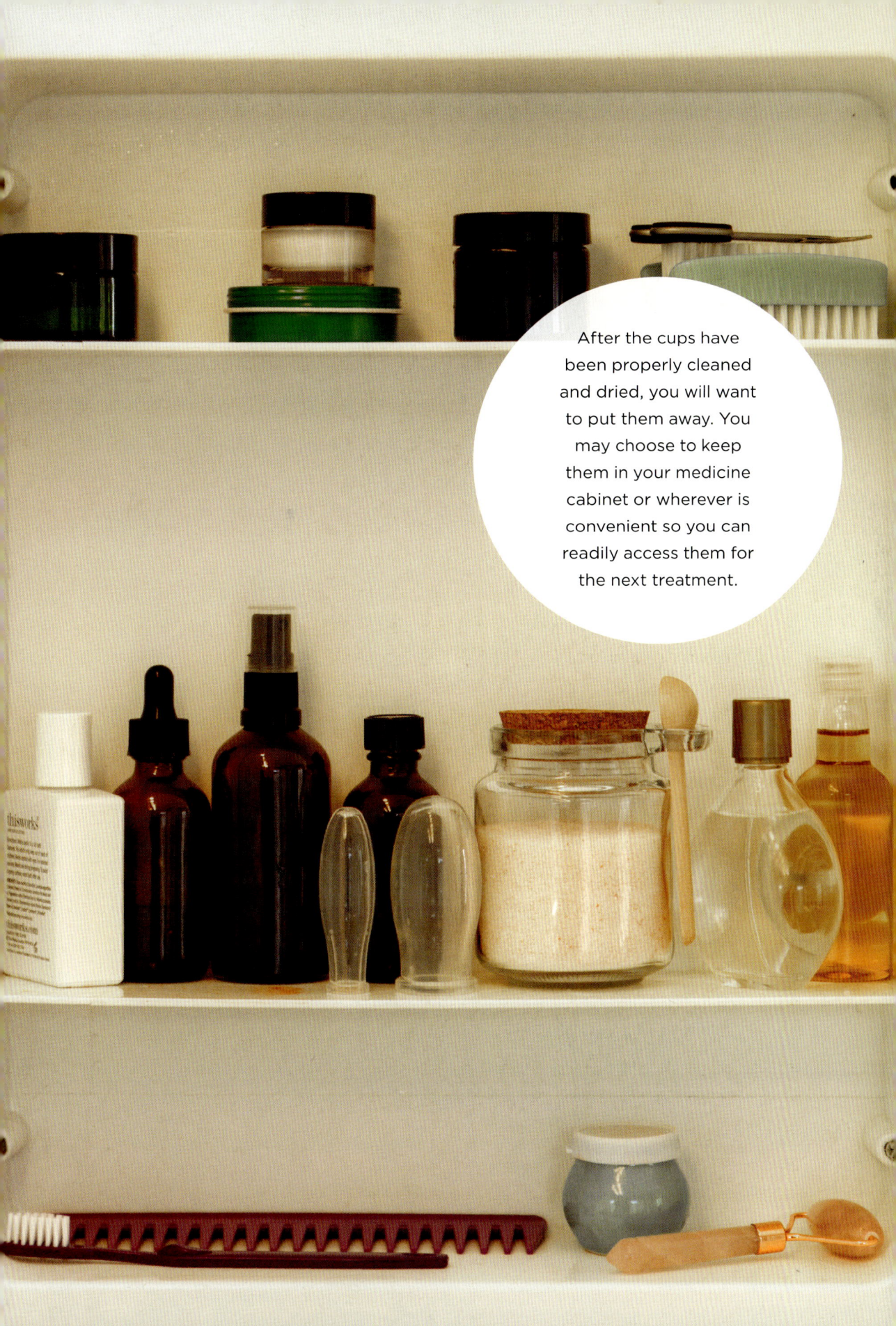

After the cups have been properly cleaned and dried, you will want to put them away. You may choose to keep them in your medicine cabinet or wherever is convenient so you can readily access them for the next treatment.

CHAPTER 4

USING CUPS ON THE FACE

Techniques for Facial Cupping
52

Methods of Application
61

**What about Cupping Marks?
(What Not to Do)**
63

Techniques for Facial Cupping

ALTHOUGH THERE are many different options for cupping for the rest of the body, facial cupping uses only two techniques: *lift-and-release* and *moving cups*. I describe both techniques below, as well as a commonly used combination of the two, which I call the *Morse Code of Cups*.

> **TREATMENT PHOTOS**
>
> The treatment photos in this book have overlays to show the direction of movement and techniques to be used.
>
> - The star marked on all cupping photos indicates the starting point(s).
>
> - Where there are arrows (any line of movement), that means you can use lift-and-release or moving cups. The arrows point in the direction of the line(s) of movement.
>
> - The Morse Code of Cups photo (on page 59) shows how lift-and-release and moving cups can be combined; this goes for any line of movement, anywhere on the face. Exceptions are the neck and delicate eye area, where only lift-and-release are used.
>
> - A few cupping treatment photos (such as the Universal Pass on page 99) have only Xs marked on them. These indicate that this treatment process uses lift-and-release only.
>
> - For the cup-free options (as on page 115), the arrows show the direction in which your fingertips will move.

LIFT-AND-RELEASE

THIS IS THE most important technique to understand. You will use it when you work down the neck, for every *Universal Pass* (see page 94), as well as in any tight or restricted areas (for many, that includes foreheads) where a moving cup simply doesn't move across smoothly.

This technique is just as its name suggests. You lift the skin with a little suction for a moment and then simply release the skin from the cup.

This gentle yet powerful technique lightly pumps the skin, stimulating microcirculation and lymphatic activity. This technique is one of the best ways to introduce cupping to the body, as it takes effect without prolonged attachment.

In many clinical settings, cupping machines offer only this lift-and-release mode for facial cupping because of how safe and effective it is. That is why this is the first thing you should learn before you move on.

The lift-and-release technique is one of the best ways to introduce cupping to the body, as it takes effect without prolonged attachment.

FAQ HOW DOES CUPPING FEEL ON THE FACE?

Cupping on the face generally feels relaxing and soothing, as well as invigorating, stimulating or warming. Often this treatment relaxes people more than they thought it would. When done correctly, it is one of the most popular facial treatments available. The one sensation you should not feel is pain — or discomfort of any kind. The cupping experience should always be a positive one.

HOW TO DO THE LIFT-AND-RELEASE TECHNIQUE

- Squeeze the cup, then lightly touch the cup to skin's surface.
- Release the squeeze of the cup while maintaining your grip on the cup.
- Gently lift the cup away from the body until you feel a slight tension engage.
- Maintain the lift hold for approximately one second.
- Then release the lift and detach the cup from the skin; squeeze the cup again to release the suction.
- Do not yank the cup off — that will hurt.
- That's it!

Try this technique on your arm or upper chest before you work on your face. Often people think they can jump right into cupping without learning the techniques first, and that is where accidents (such as cupping marks) may happen!

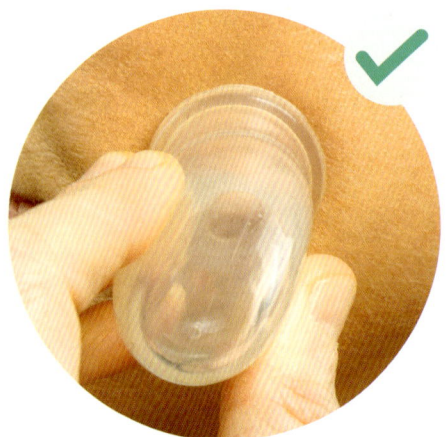

CORRECT
Lifting the cup away from your skin while cup is attached

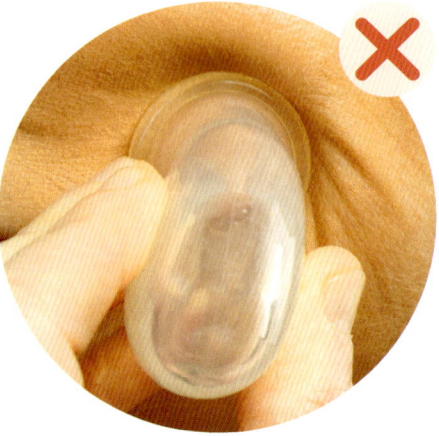

INCORRECT
Pressing the cup into your skin

HAVING A HARD TIME IMAGING THIS? Here are a few analogies that help convey this concept:

- To get the concept of application on the skin, visualize a jellyfish and the contraction (lift) and relaxation (release) of its body as it swims along.

- When manipulating the cup, think of a duck's bill quacking; mimic this like a hand puppet with the cup in your hand to get used to the squeezing and releasing of the cup.

- The lift-and-release has plunger-like effects on the body — picture the movement of a plunger (slowly and gently, though) as you use it!

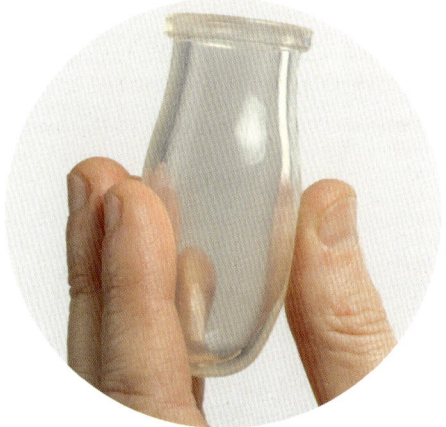

Holding the cup

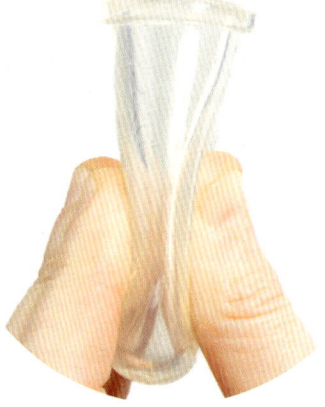

Squeezing the cup

MOVING CUPS

MOVING CUPS feel wonderful when done correctly! With every slide of the cup, you will feel the softening, toning and overall revitalizing sensation.

Imagine a vacuum cleaner (but a soothing, small and silent one), removing the lymphatic debris while you smooth out every *line of movement*. Be sure you have ample lubricant applied and do your best to make it a smooth move.

> **LINE OF MOVEMENT**
>
> *Line of movement* refers to where you move the cups in the facial cupping treatment process. Each step addresses a certain part of the face, with a starting point, a line of movement and an end point.
>
> For example, in *Step 2*, when treating *Above the Jawline*, you will attach the cup at a starting point in the middle of your chin, then move it along the jawbone, ending in front of your earlobe.

> **THREE KEYS TO ENSURING THE BEST FACIAL CUPPING**
>
> There are a few key elements that contribute to optimal facial cupping treatments: sufficient lubricant, techniques used and suction pressure.

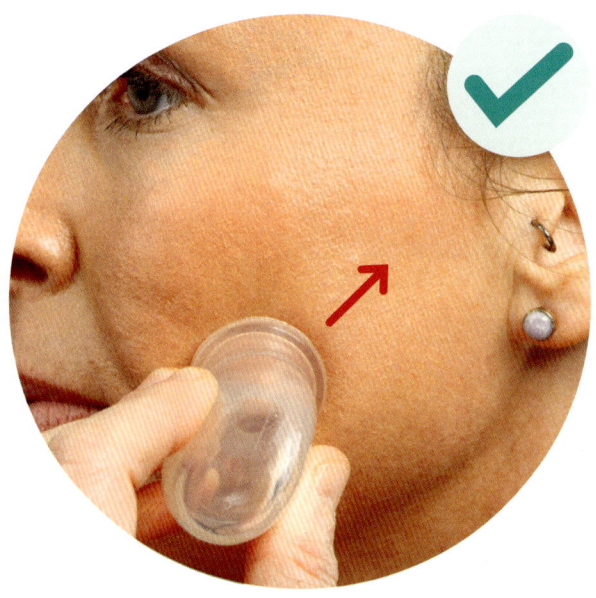

CORRECT

Sliding the cup across the skin's surface, slightly lifting the cup while still maintaining contact

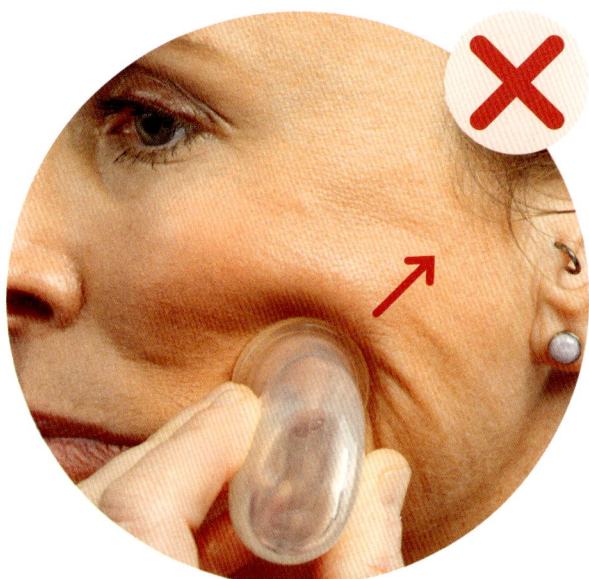

INCORRECT

Pressing the cup into your skin, trying to drag it across the face. If done incorrectly, you will notice a backup of skin in front of the cup, and the cup may be difficult to move

HOW TO DO THE MOVING CUPS TECHNIQUE

- Attach the cup to the skin using light pressure. We discuss optimal suction pressure on page 61. For now, know that each person is different, but keep the pressure light to start.

- Gently lift the cup away from the body until you feel a slight tension engage.

- While maintaining this lifted hold, slowly begin to slide the cup across the surface of your skin.

- Then release the lifted tension and release the cup from the skin by squeezing the cup again.

- Do not yank the cup off — it will hurt!

Moving cups is the most popular and easy to use technique, but many people make one common mistake: If the cup pops off at any point, they go back to the starting point and restart that line of movement. That is not correct!

That "pop off" could be a restriction (such as a tight muscle) or an anatomical "speed bump" (such as a bony ridge) that needs to be addressed where it lies. However, each line of movement needs to be finished once you have started it for optimal lymphatic efficacy. Don't overthink it; simply continue the line of movement to the end point.

So, if the cup pops off mid-movement, reattach it where it popped off and continue to the end point, using whatever technique works best. This is where what I call the Morse Code of Cups comes into play.

THE MORSE CODE OF CUPS

THE MORSE CODE OF CUPS is a combination technique of lift-and-release *and* moving cups. Once you get comfortable with the techniques and the concept of this treatment, it will become a very natural way of using the cups.

> The Morse Code is a method of communication that uses a series of dots and dashes. The *Morse Code of Cups* technique uses both the lift-and-release (dots) and moving cups (dashes).

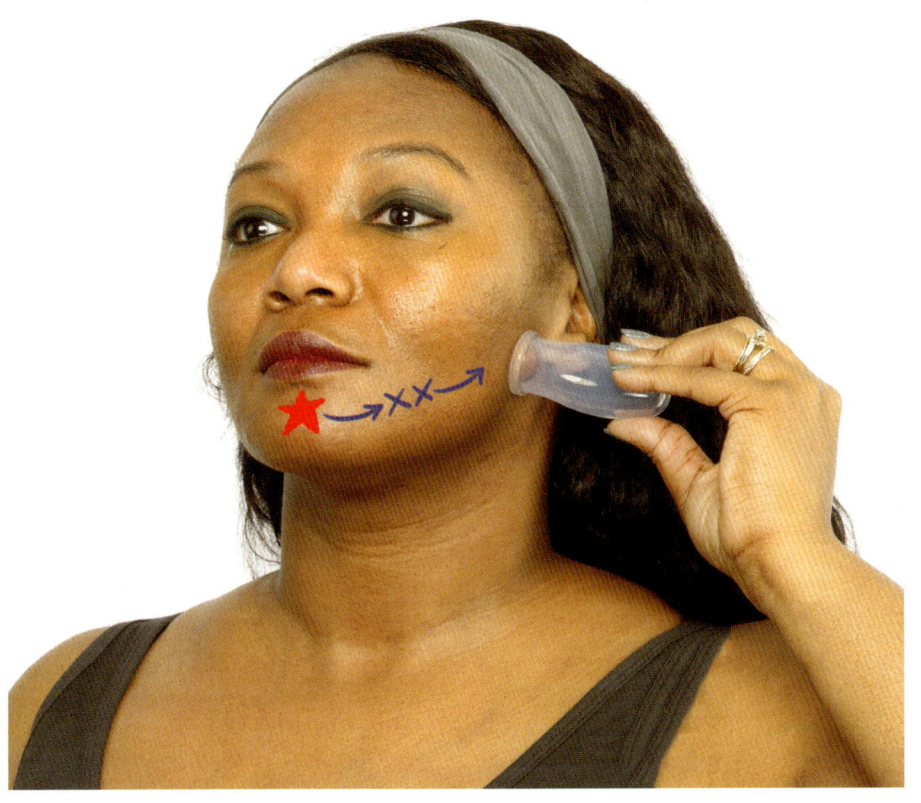

NOT SURE HOW TO CHOOSE THE BEST TECHNIQUE FOR YOUR OWN FACE?

Some people love using the moving cup everywhere possible, as it feels amazing. Others love the lift-and-release across the face, as it feels completely gentle yet stimulating every time.

Generally, you will be using a combination of the techniques — the Morse Code of Cups — across most lines of movement, so it is important to feel comfortable with both techniques.

Personally, my favorite method of application is a combination: one or two passes with the lift-and-release to pump the tissues, gently introducing the cups to every location, followed with a few passes of moving cups along the same line of movement, using the Morse Code of Cups naturally wherever needed.

See what feels best for you, what works best for your skin — and enjoy!

CUPPING AND CUP-FREE COMBINATION

There are circumstances when you may want to receive the benefits of cupping and lymph drainage, but it would be best at the time to go cup-free.

For example, perhaps the cup works at every other step of the face, but when you get to your forehead, you find it difficult to attach a cup. This may be because of muscle tension, bony ridges, prominent blood vessels or recent cosmetic injections.

If this is the case, put down the cup and use the suggested cup-free option to treat your forehead. You can try the cup another time; just do what is best for you right now for this one treatment.

For this reason, every step in this book offers cup-free options. See more about this in *Chapter 6: Before You Begin*.

Methods of Application

WHILE EVERY PERSON has a different sense of what light pressure means, it is important to acknowledge that this facial cupping treatment is meant to address the most superficial layers of soft tissue in the face.

SUCTION PRESSURE SHOULD ALWAYS BE LIGHT

That means there is no need to use strong suction pressure! Do your best to use lighter pressure for this treatment, as it works every time and yields all the amazing results we discuss.

When I'm teaching cupping, I tell students to remember this saying: *If you want to keep the skin tight, you have to make sure the suction pressure is light!*

The good news is that most silicone face cups have a "maximum" suction when you squeeze them, and that maximum is safe for facial cupping, so you don't need to be too afraid.

I recommend testing the suction pressure on your upper chest or arm before you approach your face. First, try squeezing the cup a little — not squeezing it as much as possible — and attaching it to your skin to see how it feels. Then squeeze it all the way so you feel the difference.

> Even with silicone cups, be sure to use whatever lighter pressure moves easily and feels the best for your skin.

MOVEMENTS ARE SLOWER, RHYTHMIC AND REPETITIVE

- **SLOWER PACE.** Any technique you use should be applied slowly across the face — nothing too fast or vigorous. Fast or vigorous movements could irritate the delicate skin of the face and are not as effective as movements made at a nice, relaxed pace. The movements shouldn't be too slow, either. Just go with a smooth, even pace. *The entire treatment process should take approximately 15 to 20 minutes.*

- **RHYTHMIC APPLICATION.** Once you get the hang of it, try to maintain an easy, rhythmic pace so you create a uniform application over every section and over the entire face. Especially when working down the front of the neck, a slower, rhythmic pace ensures all the nerves and circulatory vessels remain undisturbed.

- **REPETITIVE MOVEMENTS.** As with most types of bodywork, repetition is necessary for both efficacy and general feel-good benefit. Think about it: one pass over the area is considered an introduction; two passes will get things moving; three to five passes will really complete the process beautifully! Still, do not overdo it. After years of practical applications, I've found that three to five passes is best for all faces.

What about Cupping Marks?
(WHAT NOT TO DO)

OH, THE MILLION-DOLLAR question of cupping marks. One of the most common questions I hear about facial cupping is about those eye-catching, bruise-resembling cupping marks potentially appearing on the face.

While cupping marks are common responses to stronger, more clinical applications on other parts of the body, there are many therapeutic benefits available from cups that do not mark the skin at all, especially in this facial cupping treatment.

Obviously, when you are doing facial cupping for cosmetic purposes, cupping marks are to be avoided. For this reason, the facial cupping techniques recommended here are the only methods of application that you should use.

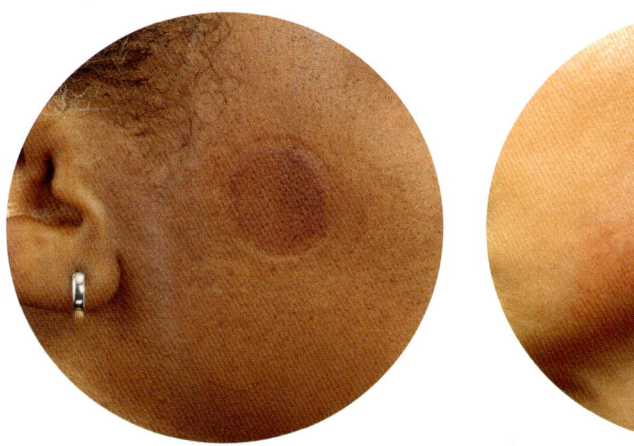
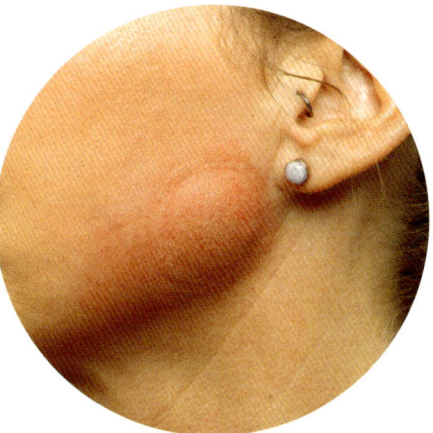

Additionally, watching yourself in the mirror as you do this treatment will allow you to see how your skin is responding and you can adjust as needed.

For example, one of the primary indications to stop cupping an area is if the skin starts to get red. While some pinkness to the skin is welcome — it indicates stimulated blood flow — redness can indicate overstimulation of the capillaries in the dermis, resulting in vascular microtraumas, which can cause those cupping marks.

WHAT NOT TO DO

- **DO NOT USE INSUFFICIENT LUBRICATION.** This is the first thing to check before you begin, because it is that important for ensuring optimal treatment. Using a cup on drier skin will likely result in cupping marks.

- **DO NOT USE STRONG SUCTION PRESSURE.** Lighter pressure is all you need for facial cupping. Every person should use lighter, easy-to-move suction pressure to avoid cupping marks on the face. Strong pressure not only makes it hard to move the cup, it could also easily cause cupping marks.

- **DO NOT USE AN INAPPROPRIATE CUP SIZE.** Size matters for facial cupping. Use the largest cup available for any location. A large cup will safely address more surface tissue for greatest efficacy, dispersing suction pressure more evenly across the area. For example, you have to use your smallest cup in the upper lip region but using your smallest cup across the cheek may result in cupping marks, so be sure to switch to a larger cup for the cheek.

- **DO NOT FORCE A MOVING CUP.** At any location where your moving cup meets resistance, there is a reason to stop. It could be not enough lubrication, or a tight muscle or a bony ridge in your face. Check lubrication, or simply revert to lift-and-release over these areas to avoid cupping marks.

- **DO NOT USE STATIONARY CUPS.** For this facial cupping treatment, there is no reason to park a cup anywhere. Stationary cups are known for being able to leave cupping marks.

- **DO NOT OVERWORK AN AREA.** If you do too much cupping across the same line of movement, chances are high that the skin will begin to show cupping marks. For this reason, three to five passes over every line of movement are best. While a warm glow is optimal and normal (due to the increased blood flow), if the skin becomes red, stop cupping that area. Also, don't overwork wrinkled areas. Cupping is known to release tension in muscles, which can result in cupping marks. If you travel across tight, wrinkled areas (such as the forehead or jaw area), anything more than the recommended three to five passes could result in cupping marks.

WHAT IF YOU *DO* GET CUPPING MARKS?

One of the reasons this book came to be is because so many people were doing facial cupping incorrectly.

While you are unlikely to get cupping marks if all suggestions have been followed, any cupping marks should not cause much alarm. Cupping marks fade within a few days at the most, and your skin will look as it did before without any adverse changes.

While cupping marks are not bruises, they look like them, therefore your skin will take a few days to process these cupping marks in a way similar to how your body takes a few days to process a bruise. Additionally, the face is highly vascularized (meaning there is a high concentration of blood and lymph vessels), so the process of dissolving the cupping mark will happen quickly.

If you do make a mistake, your skin will recover without issue.

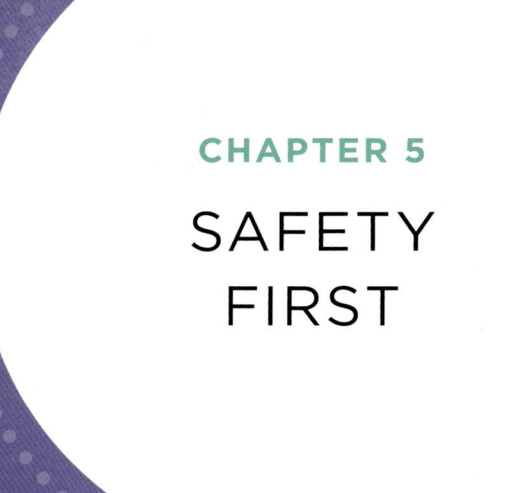

CHAPTER 5

SAFETY FIRST

Endangerment Sites
68

Working with Cosmetic Injections
72

Post-Surgical Considerations
73

WHEN USING CUPS on the face and neck, it is very important to understand some key safety points before you get started. In this chapter we look at cupping safely, specifically as related to endangerment sites, cosmetic injections and any recent surgical procedures.

Endangerment Sites

THERE ARE LOCATIONS on the body called *endangerment sites*. These locations require a cautious approach when it comes to cupping. They contain nerves, blood and lymph vessels that are closer to the surface, making them more vulnerable to damage with any bodywork or cupping.

Here, we are concerned about the endangerment sites related to the face and neck.

ANTERIOR TRIANGLE

THE FRONT OF THE NECK — from ear to ear, jawline to collarbones — contains one of the body's most vulnerable endangerment sites, generally referred to as the *anterior triangle*. This region contains many vital blood vessels, lymph nodes and nerves. It should therefore be approached with a lot of caution when doing facial cupping.

The only technique to use in this region is the lift-and-release and using light suction pressure only. Never using moving cups and never use strong suction pressure here. Any suction that is too strong or movements that are too vigorous could harm the delicate anatomy located in the front of the neck. I often refer to this region as a "no-slide zone."

You will travel down through this area many times during the treatment, though, since it is important to stimulate all the lymph nodes located throughout this region and in the direction instructed.

At the beginning of *Chapter 7: Facial Cupping Step-By-Step Treatment*, you will learn how to safely work through this area. We will identify the exact line of movement down the neck, and the "jump-off" location from the face where you will always return to lift-and-release along the specified, exact line of movement through this endangerment site.

While some may think cupping through here is unsafe, I assure you that when you follow the guidelines outlined in *Chapter 7* — with or without a cup — everything will be perfectly safe and very effective.

> **ANATOMY FYI**
>
> The front of the neck is commonly called the anterior triangle, but technically there are two triangulated sections of vulnerable anatomy here: the *posterior triangle* and the *anterior triangle*.
>
> They are generally referred to as the anterior triangle due to their location at the front of the neck, as "anterior" means closer to the front.

ENDANGERMENT SITES AT THE FRONT OF NECK

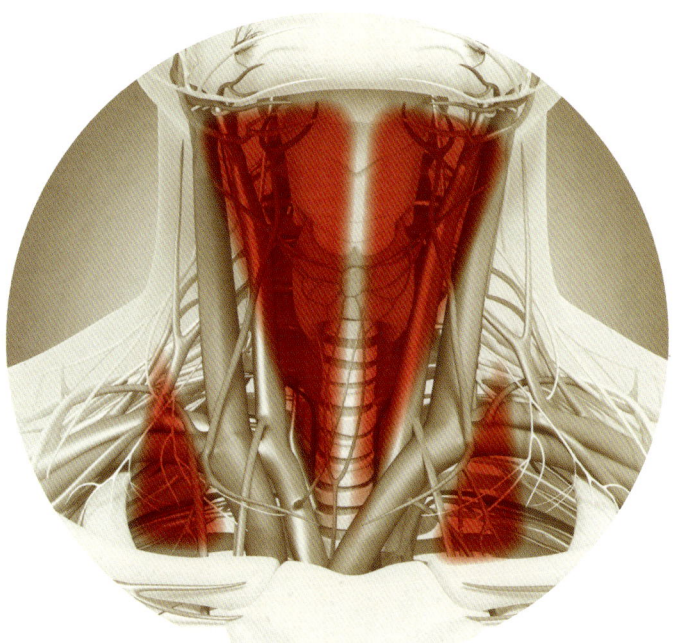

The anterior and posterior triangles, marked here, are endangerment sites and collectively known as the anterior triangle.

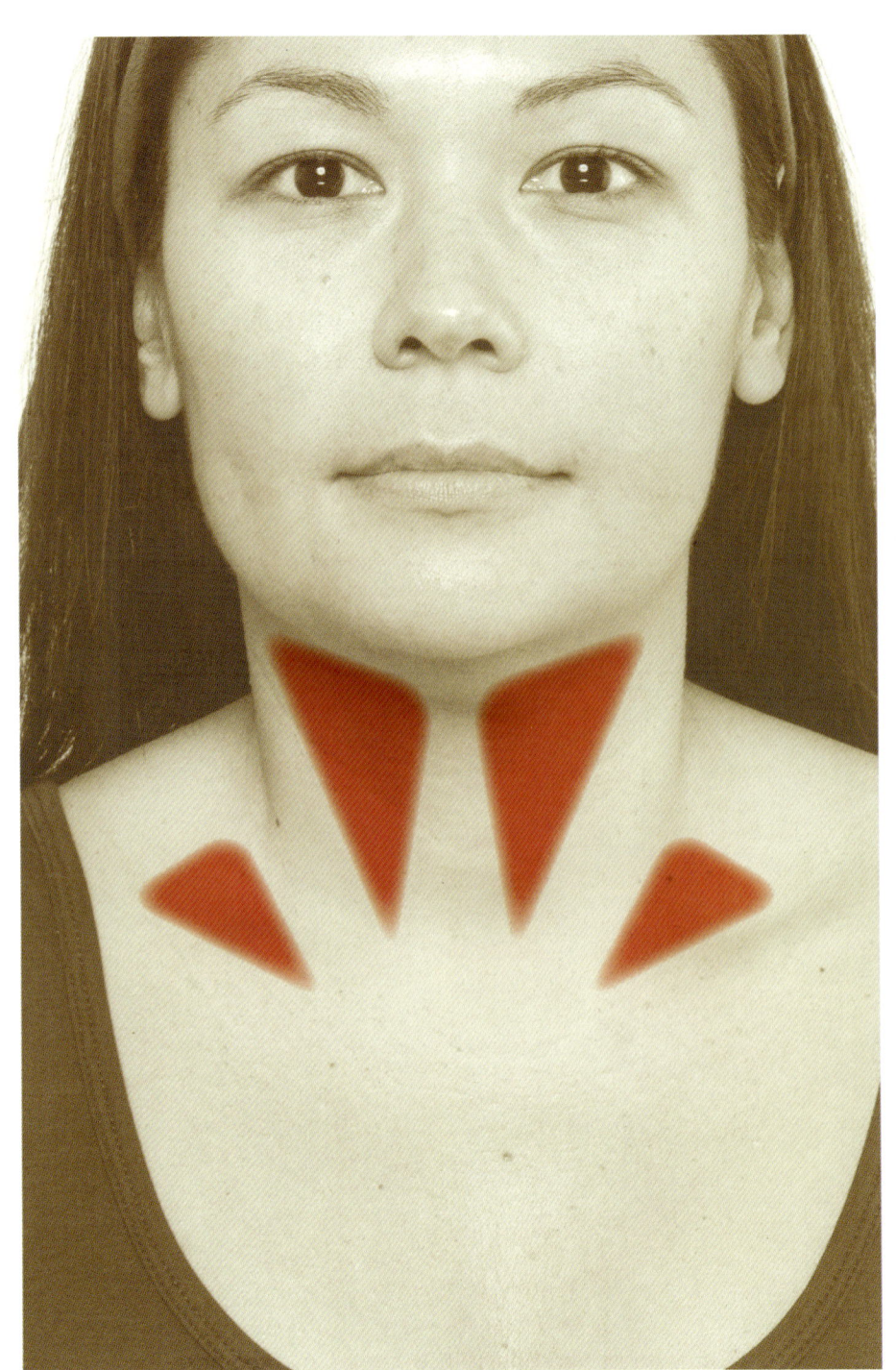

You will learn how to safely work through the area of the anterior triangle at the beginning of *Chapter 7: Facial Cupping Step-by-Step Treatment*.

TEMPORAL REGION

LOCATED BETWEEN the hairline and the outside edges of the eyes is the small endangerment site known as the *temporal region*, commonly called the temple area or temples.

There are important blood vessels and nerves located here, so caution should be used when working through this area, too. Sometimes, you can actually see blue-colored veins in this region and, if you have ever had a headache, you might naturally feel compelled to massage this area.

Every person has different skin, some thinner or more fragile than others; in this region, blood vessels may protrude on some people while on others they are barely visible. If you have veins that bulge here, detach the cup as you approach the area — in *Step 4* for the forehead and *Step 5* for the eyes — and skip over them, then reattach the cup and continue the line of movement.

Again, to keep the treatment safe and comfortable, do not use any stronger suction pressure here, and skip over any prominent blood vessels in this common endangerment site.

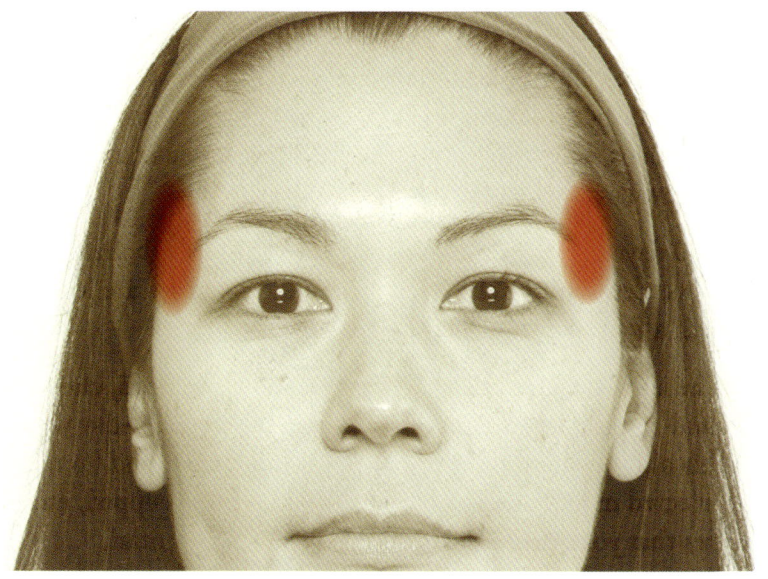

The temporal region, marked here, is another endangerment site.

Working with Cosmetic Injections

COSMETIC INJECTIONS are widely available today for many different cosmetically focused reasons. However, with facial cupping there are specific safety considerations to acknowledge.

If any materials have been injected into the face area, you should avoid working over the entire face for approximately 30 days. This goes for any fillers or wrinkle-fighting materials.

Why? The material that has been injected is intended to stay exactly where it is. If you attempt to use cups over the area, these materials will be dislodged from their intended locations and begin to travel along lymph drainage pathways to other locations. For example, Botox is a modified neurotoxic protein that is intended to stay where it has been applied in order to block nerve conduction to a muscle, thus inhibiting muscle contractions that cause wrinkles.

While a neurotoxin is generally safe wherever it is injected, if it enters the circulation, it could cause muscle weakness, nausea, vision problems, trouble speaking or swallowing, breathing problems or loss of bladder control. Any other injected materials (collagen, fat transfers, etc.) that are meant for cosmetic enhancement are also injected with location-specific intentions, so if you use cups too soon then you could move those materials elsewhere in the body.

After 30 days, the injected materials have been metabolized and thoroughly settled into the site of application, so chances are less that cupping will affect their intended usage.

Just to be sure, travel over the area in question (forehead, cheeks, etc.) with lift-and-release only for that first session after the 30-day waiting period. This allows you to test how the local tissues respond (to make sure the injected materials don't irritate the skin when cupped, etc.) and ensures that your tissue isn't too sensitive for this initial, post-injection treatment.

Post-Surgical Considerations

WHETHER YOU'VE HAD a small eyelid lift or a full facelift, any surgical interventions should be left to fully heal for at least six to eight weeks before you attempt any cupping over or around the area.

Further, no cupping should ever be done if there remain any scabs, sutures, significant bruising or raw tissue, as these are clear indications that the area is still healing and is too fragile for cupping.

Often, I encourage people who are having such surgical procedures to receive medical release from their surgeon to receive facial cupping. If their surgeon is not familiar with this manner of cupping, then asking for medical release to receive an "invigorating face massage" will suffice.

If there is a question or concern of safe timing, please do not attempt any face cupping just yet! Over the years we have found that it is better to wait slightly longer and be sure, rather than possibly hinder or delay the healing process. Additionally, consider finding a professionally trained facial cupping person for that first treatment post-surgery if any questions remain.

CHAPTER 6

BEFORE YOU BEGIN

Assessing Your Skin
76

Exceptions and What-Ifs
77

Preparing for Facial Cupping
84

Know Your Limits and When to Seek Professional Assistance
87

Assessing Your Skin

IN PREPARATION for facial cupping, it is important to take personal inventory and thoroughly examine your skin to create the best treatment plan.

- Is your skin dry? The average skin type requires approximately a coin-sized amount of oil to have a successful outcome. If the skin is naturally hydrated, the moving cups will slide across the skin easily. But if your skin is dry and dehydrated, you will need a little more oil than others.

- Is your skin loose along the jawline? At first, a moving cup will not move easily, so you will have to use lift-and-release more over these areas until the toning improves in subsequent treatments.

- Are there any protruding veins around your temples? You will have to skip over the protruding veins with the cup.

- Do you have raised moles or skin tags? Avoid moving cups across them, as it will hurt or possibly tear your skin; use lift-and-release instead to address them as you move through the area.

- Do you have acne issues? Facial hair? Jaw muscle tension?

This section will address many common exceptions which, if they apply to you, will require you to personalize the standard treatment process.

There are also many conditions that affect the facial skin a little more dramatically than others, such as rosacea. If your skin's needs are more complicated than the exceptions listed here, consider seeking professional facial cupping services before you take on your own self-care. For more information, see *Know Your Limits* on page 87.

> **SAFETY POINT:** Do not attempt facial cupping if any infectious or contagious conditions are present. If you have any infection, from cold sores to impetigo, avoid treating your face completely and wait until the skin has cleared before you begin facial cupping treatment.

Exceptions and What-Ifs

CUP-FREE OPTIONS

FOR EVERY STEP of the cupping treatment, I have also recommended cup-free options.

It is important to address the entire face every time, so be sure not to skip any section of your face if the skin does not respond easily to the general cupping instructions. Considering the major role of lymph drainage in this facial cupping treatment, the recommended cup-free options will be your best way to address any area where a cup cannot be used without excluding it from the treatment.

You will do the cup-free options with your hands instead of cups. For most of the cup-free options, your fingers will be flattened and closed together, making contact with as much surface area as possible.

If choosing these cup-free options, be sure to follow them as instructed for each step; the cup-free options follow manual lymph drainage techniques as done in a general facial treatment.

WHAT IF ... FACIAL HAIR?

HERE WE ARE referring to thicker, more coarse facial hair such as beards and mustaches, not the hair that naturally exists on the surface of all skin. When this type of facial hair is present, it can make it difficult to create the sealed connection between the cup and the skin's surface, especially if trying to use the lighter suction pressure required for facial cupping.

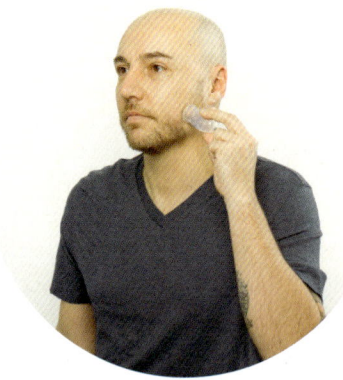 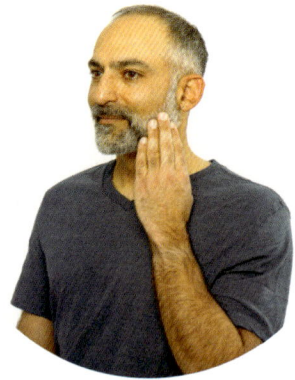

With shorter or thinner facial hair, it may be possible to attach a cup. With thicker or more coarse facial hair, using the cup-free option works best.

While it is possible to cup over some body hair, facial hair has many variations, and you need to consider these when deciding if cups will work or not. Has it been shaved recently? Then the cups may attach without issue. Is it a full beard or a mustache? Cups will not attach over beards or mustaches of any length. Is the hair thin and soft or thick and coarse? If shorter, more recently shaved or more sparse facial hair, with an ample amount of applied oil, it may allow for some lift-and-release or perhaps even some moving cups. On the other hand, longer or thicker facial hair will not allow for a cup to attach at all.

Assess your facial hair according to these suggestions; perhaps try to attach a cup (without force) and then decide if you can proceed with cups or not.

Eyebrows need to be addressed differently on an individual basis, too. The hair varies tremendously from person to person. A thinner eyebrow is easily cupped, while a thicker eyebrow cannot be cupped at all.

Do not just skip over any hair-covered areas. It is important to address the entire face. There is a wealth of lymphatic activity over every area of the face, especially along the jawline and lower cheeks, where facial hair commonly grows. Using the cup-free options will ensure optimal results for the entire face.

RECOMMENDATION: Use your fingertips to follow the cup-free recommendations, which are described for every step of the treatment process.

WHAT IF ... ACNE?

ACNE IS a dermatological condition that affects a great number of people. Acne is characterized by inflamed or infected sebaceous glands in the skin, most identified by red pimples and blemishes on the face. Acne commonly affects hormonal teenagers, but it can also occur for many other reasons, such as poor diet, environmental exposure or inadequate skincare.

While cupping may help clear the congestion associated with non-hormonal acne, it is important to work mindfully around pimples and acne spots. Try avoiding them and do your best not to "pop" them while you work, since that would create an open wound, which in turn could allow either blood to escape or bacteria to enter the skin.

If by chance you pop a pimple, be sure to clean the skin's surface immediately and thoroughly clean the cup, too. Never continue the treatment over the popped pimple, as that is now an open wound.

RECOMMENDATION: If you approach a pimple as you work, employ the lift-and-release technique to skip over that spot. If an area has many acne spots, consider using the cup-free options until the breakout has cleared.

WHAT IF ... SINUS CONGESTION?

FACE CUPPING has many wonderful benefits, and relieving the congestion associated with sinus issues is one of the most popular!

There are several locations in the face and head that are more affected when sinus congestion is a consideration, specifically around the nose, cheeks and forehead. As you work through each of these affected areas, you may encounter some sensitive locations if sinus congestion is an issue. If yes, be sure to work with comfort in mind and follow the recommendations accordingly.

RECOMMENDATION: Use the lift-and-release technique over any hypersensitive or congested areas.

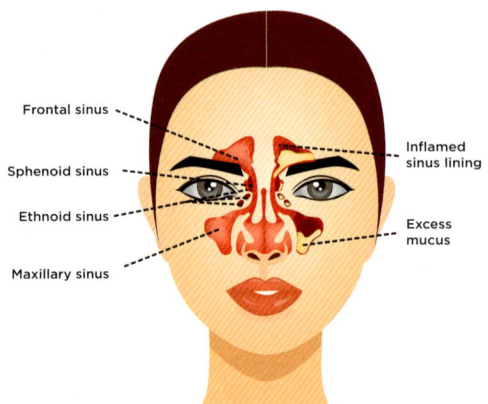
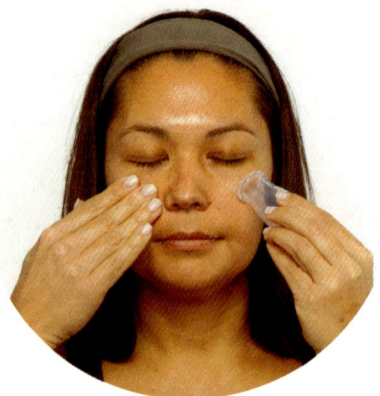

FAQ CAN I DO THIS FACIAL CUPPING TREATMENT WHEN I HAVE A COLD OR FLU?

Do *not* do this treatment within the first 72 hours of onset of sickness. Why? When you start feeling ill, your lymphatic system is working hard to produce immune-fighting cells to rush into the sinus areas and fight the infecting sickness. If you clear this necessary excess of lymph fluids, your body will be forced to work even harder to replace what you cleared with the cups.

After the first 72 hours, chances are you can proceed without issue — and feel better fast! Please practice safety first and wait the 72 hours before clearing this type of sinus congestion.

WHAT IF ... JAW TENSION?

OFTEN, YOU WILL encounter resistance as you travel across the middle of your jawbone and cheek where the muscles of your jaw attach.

If you suffer from TMJ dysfunction, this will be even more obvious. This area holds a lot of muscular tension, as the mighty masseter muscle involved with the movements of the jaw has attachment sites in these regions. Additionally, muscles around the mouth that contribute to wrinkles can receive great tension release from treating this area.

Cupping along this line of movement can release muscular tension, alleviate TMJD discomfort and reduce wrinkle patterns.

RECOMMENDATION: If you encounter any "speed bumps" along the way, do not force the cup to move across it. Instead, simply revert to the lift-and-release technique to get across that section. Thereafter, you can finish that line of movement with another moving cup, employing the Morse Code of Cups combination technique (see page 59) or simply finish that line of movement with lift-and-release.

Note: If you try to work through the tension too forcefully, a cupping mark could appear! For more information on how to avoid cupping marks on the face, see pages 64–65.

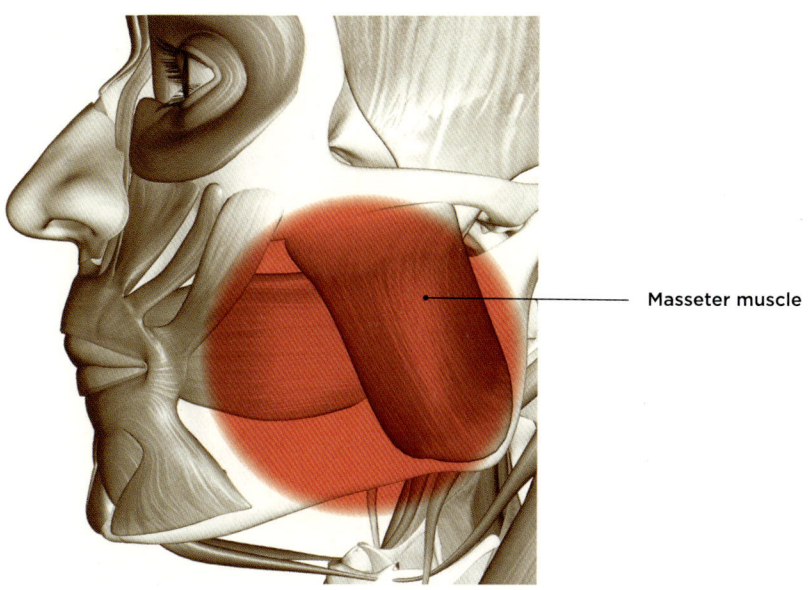

Masseter muscle

WHAT IF ... VERY LOOSE SKIN?

LOOSE FACIAL SKIN can occur for many reasons and can affect any region of the face, the most common areas being along the jawline.

If excessively loose skin does not allow for an easy-to-slide moving cup, follow the recommendations here so you can treat your entire face without skipping any areas.

RECOMMENDATION: Use the lift-and-release technique to address the line of movement across areas of very loose skin. With time and later treatments, the tissue's tonicity will tighten up, indicating improvement, which will progressively allow for smooth moving cups and safe tissue-toning.

WHAT IF ... RECENT COSMETIC PROCEDURES?

TODAY, THERE ARE many options for people seeking the assistance of professional cosmetic enhancements. And while facial cupping is still great to do no matter what procedure you've had, it is important to proceed with timing and caution in mind for your best outcome.

For more details about injections and surgical procedures, please revisit *Chapter 5: Safety First*, where both scenarios are detailed. Since there are major differences between injections and surgical procedures, they are addressed independently here.

INJECTIONS?

Regardless of the material injected, wait approximately 30 days before attempting this facial cupping treatment. Why? After 30 days, the injected materials have been metabolized and settled into the site of application, so chances are less that cupping will affect their intended usage.

RECOMMENDATION: After 30 days, use lift-and-release only across the sites of injections during that first treatment. If your skin is sensitive to that technique, switch to cup-free options for these areas. At the next treatment (a few days later or thereafter), try lift-and-release again and, if not sensitive, proceed with whichever technique you prefer.

> **SAFETY NOTE:** If you have any other concerns beyond what is mentioned here, always check with the medical professional who did the injections. Ask if you can receive an "invigorating face massage." Why? Although facial cupping is becoming more popular, not all medical professionals are familiar with this manner of cupping and its effects on the skin, muscles and circulation. Therefore, asking for medical approval to receive an "invigorating face massage" will address the same concerns.

COSMETIC SURGERY?

No matter what the surgical procedure, the skin, circulatory system and muscles have all been affected and need time to heal. The minimum waiting time post-surgical procedure is six to eight weeks. Post-surgery procedures were discussed in *Chapter 5: Safety Concerns*, so please review that information if needed.

RECOMMENDATION: When the time comes, use lift-and-release only for the first treatment to test how your skin will respond, especially close to any site of incision. If there are any areas that are sensitive or uncomfortable, switch to the cup-free recommendations until things feel better. It takes time to heal and, while it may be frustrating, it is in your best interest to wait until your skin is ready.

> **SAFETY NOTE:** Still have questions? Please check with your cosmetic surgeon for when you can receive facial cupping or an "invigorating face massage," as mentioned above. Also consider working with a trained professional for that first facial cupping treatment to get you started in the right direction.

Preparing for Facial Cupping

AS YOU GET READY for the facial cupping treatment, it is important to prepare your skin accordingly. While cleansing your face is not required, it is highly recommended.

Yes, you can work over makeup, but since you need oil to do the cupping, things could get messy, both on the surface of your skin as well as the surface of the cup. Additionally, your pores will be open and skin will be ready for great products to be applied thereafter.

Start with a clean face for the best results.

CONSIDER A WARMING OPTION. Adding any warming treatment will further soften your skin before you begin. Use a steam towel or perhaps a warm shower or bath to cleanse and soften the skin. Facial steaming treatments are great as a pretreatment option, too. Warm face tissue will also help to facilitate smoother moving cups, as the skin, muscles and fascia have been softened.

WORK IN FRONT OF A MIRROR. You will want to work in front of a mirror, either standing or sitting, whatever your preference. Using a mirror helps you watch where you are working as you follow along with the step-by-step images in the next chapter. Working with a mirror especially helps you monitor any tissue responses that might indicate the need to change the treatment. Remember that while some pinkness is good, redness means it is either too strong or too much treatment over the area. Also, you will enjoy watching your face's reaction to the treatment, as your skin will liven up immediately. It's quite entertaining to watch the process!

DON'T FORGET THE FACE OIL. As I've mentioned several times now, oil is a crucial component to a successful outcome. No matter the choice, be sure to have the oil with you and apply it generously before you begin. Choose your favorite oil for the treatment, have a small hand towel nearby to wipe your hands off after you apply the oil to your skin and get the cups ready.

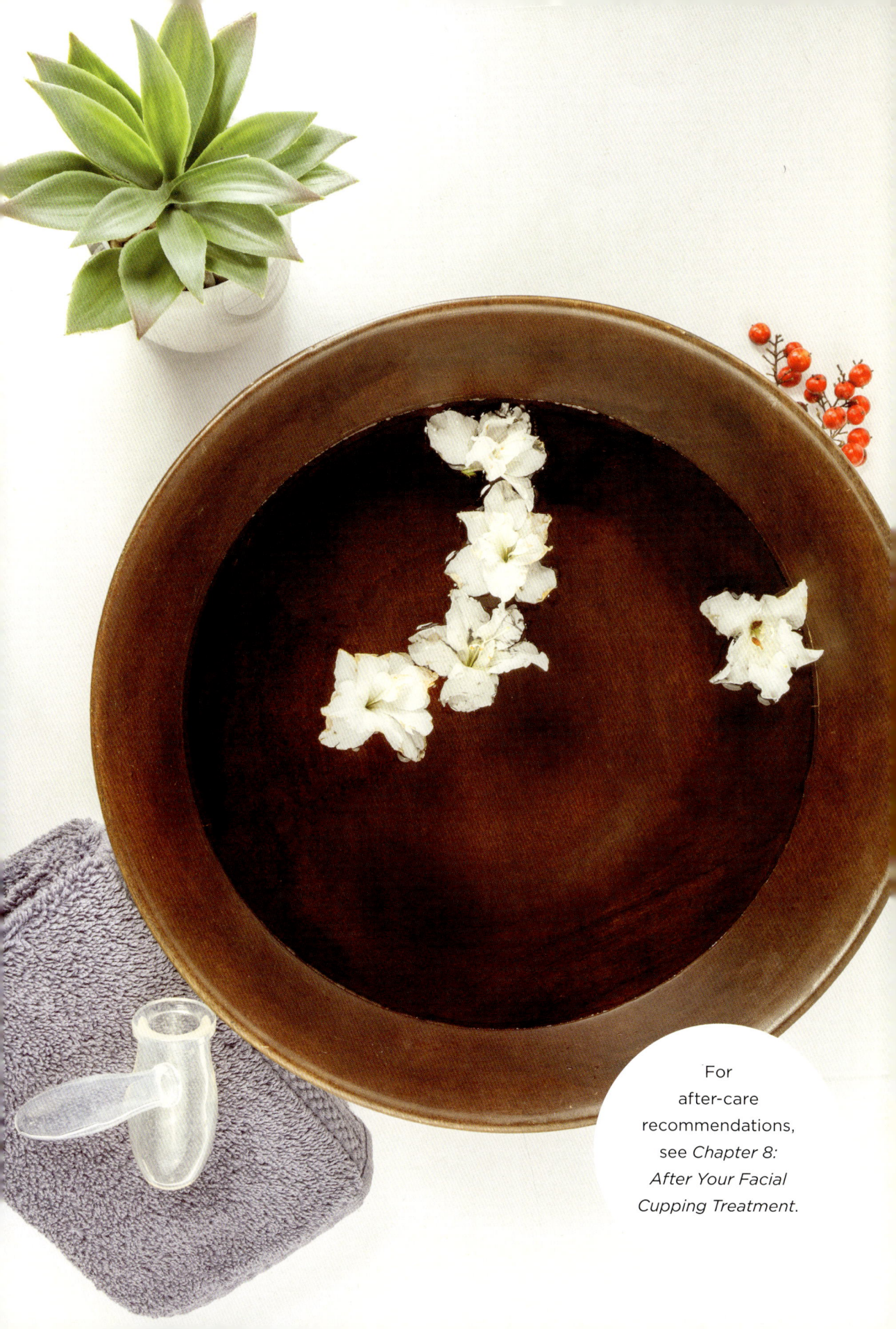

For after-care recommendations, see *Chapter 8: After Your Facial Cupping Treatment*.

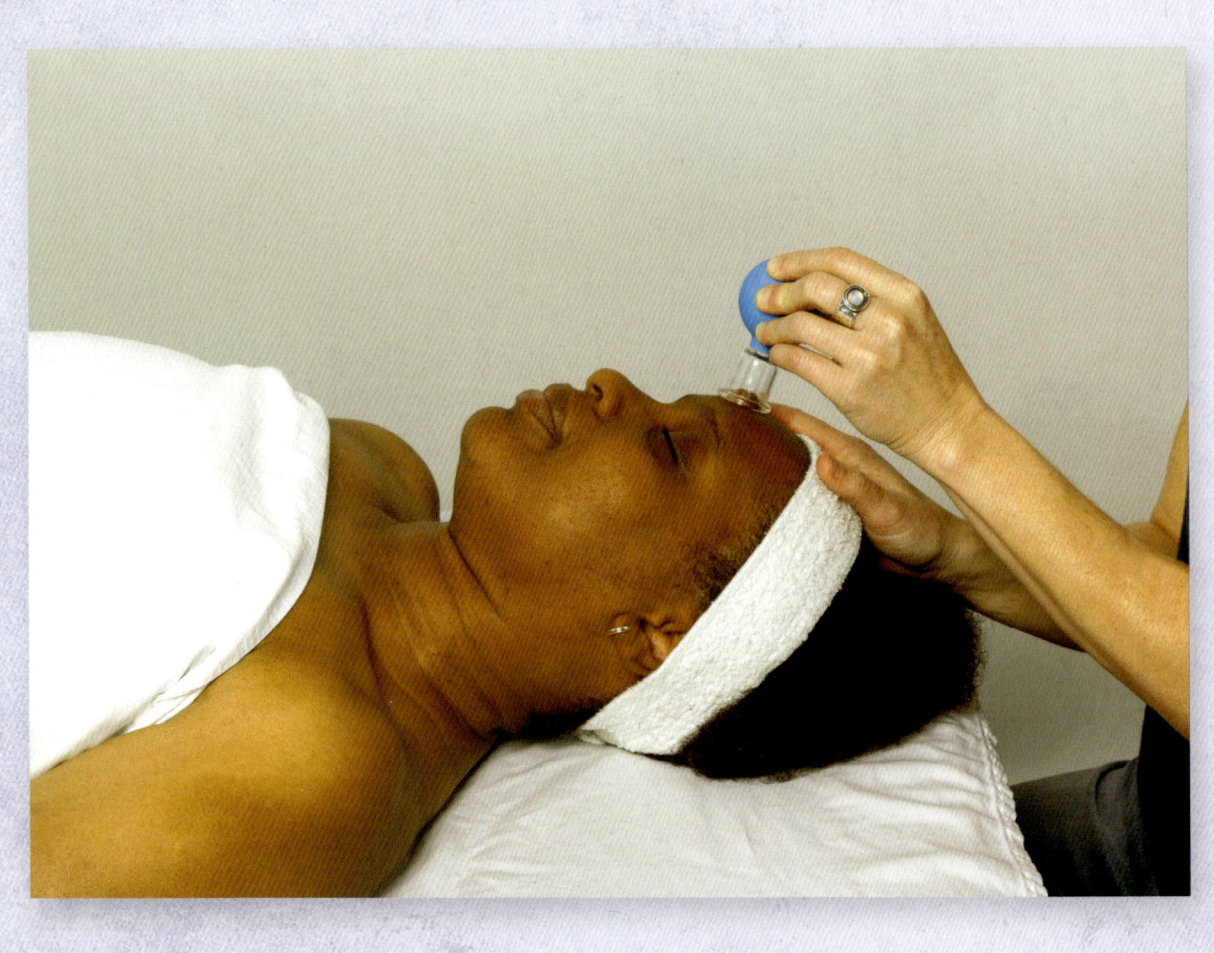

Know Your Limits and When to Seek Professional Assistance

THERE ARE SO MANY benefits that can be had from facial cupping. However, there are many skin or medical conditions that would be best served by professional assessment and treatment rather than by self-care.

Many dermatological skin conditions such as rosacea, dermatitis and cystic acne require a professional's insight for the best treatment. Other medically involved conditions such as Bell's palsy, trigeminal neuralgia or any type of facial reconstruction procedure can also receive amazing benefit from facial cupping, but each of those conditions requires a great deal of clinical expertise.

While the benefit of facial cupping is all-encompassing for face skin health, the methods of applications for more complex conditions are beyond the scope of this book. If you and your skin require special attention beyond the suggestions made in this book, please honor the process and respect the limits of self-care discussed here.

I promise you will enjoy facial cupping for self-care when the time is right and your face is ready.

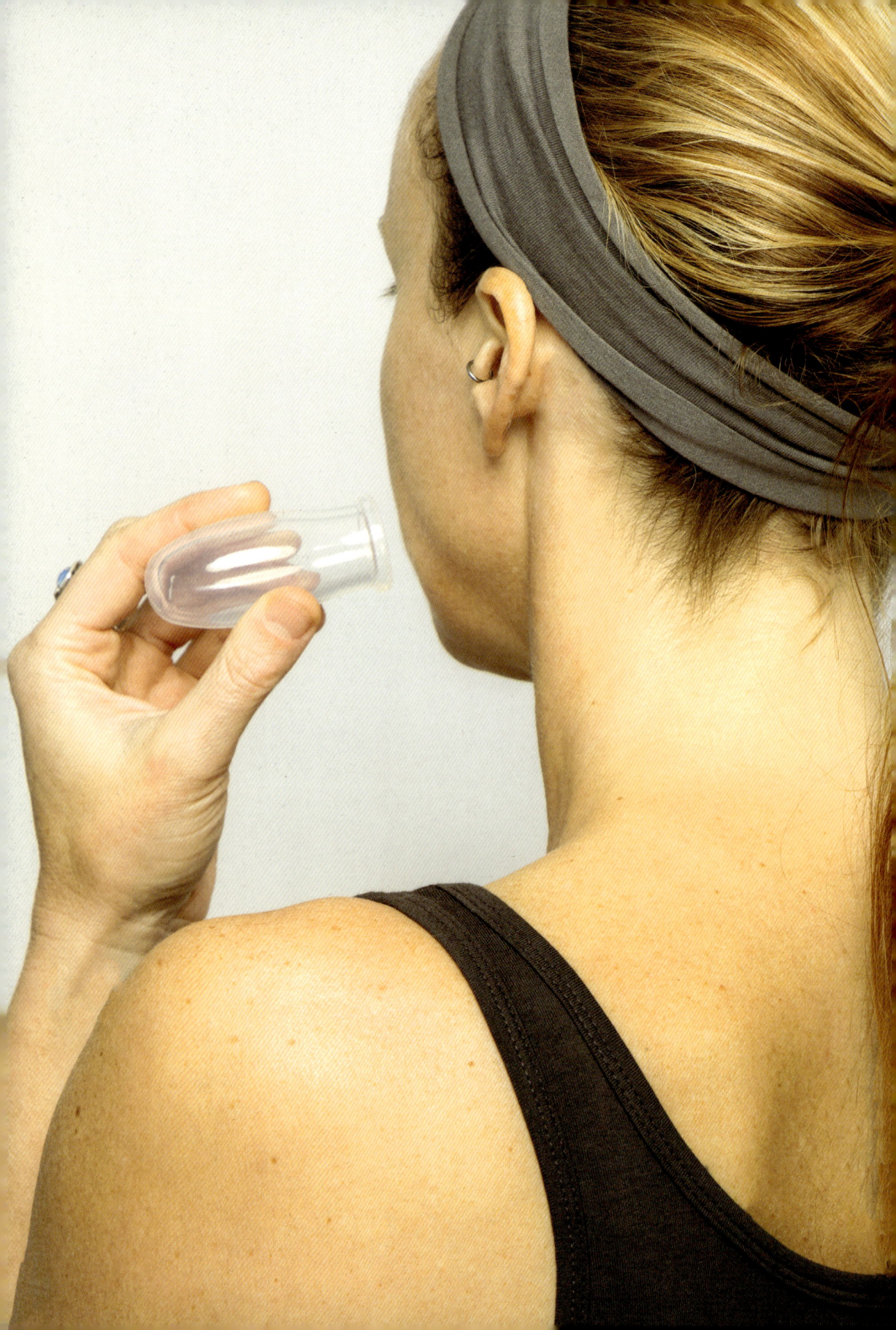

CHAPTER 7

FACIAL CUPPING STEP-BY-STEP TREATMENT

Overview of Treatment Process 91

Understanding the Universal Pass 94

Step 1: The Neck and Upper Chest 105

Step 2: The Jawline 111

Step 3: The Cheeks and Upper Lip 121

Step 4: The Forehead 131

Step 5: The Eye Area 141

The Face-Cupping Map 150

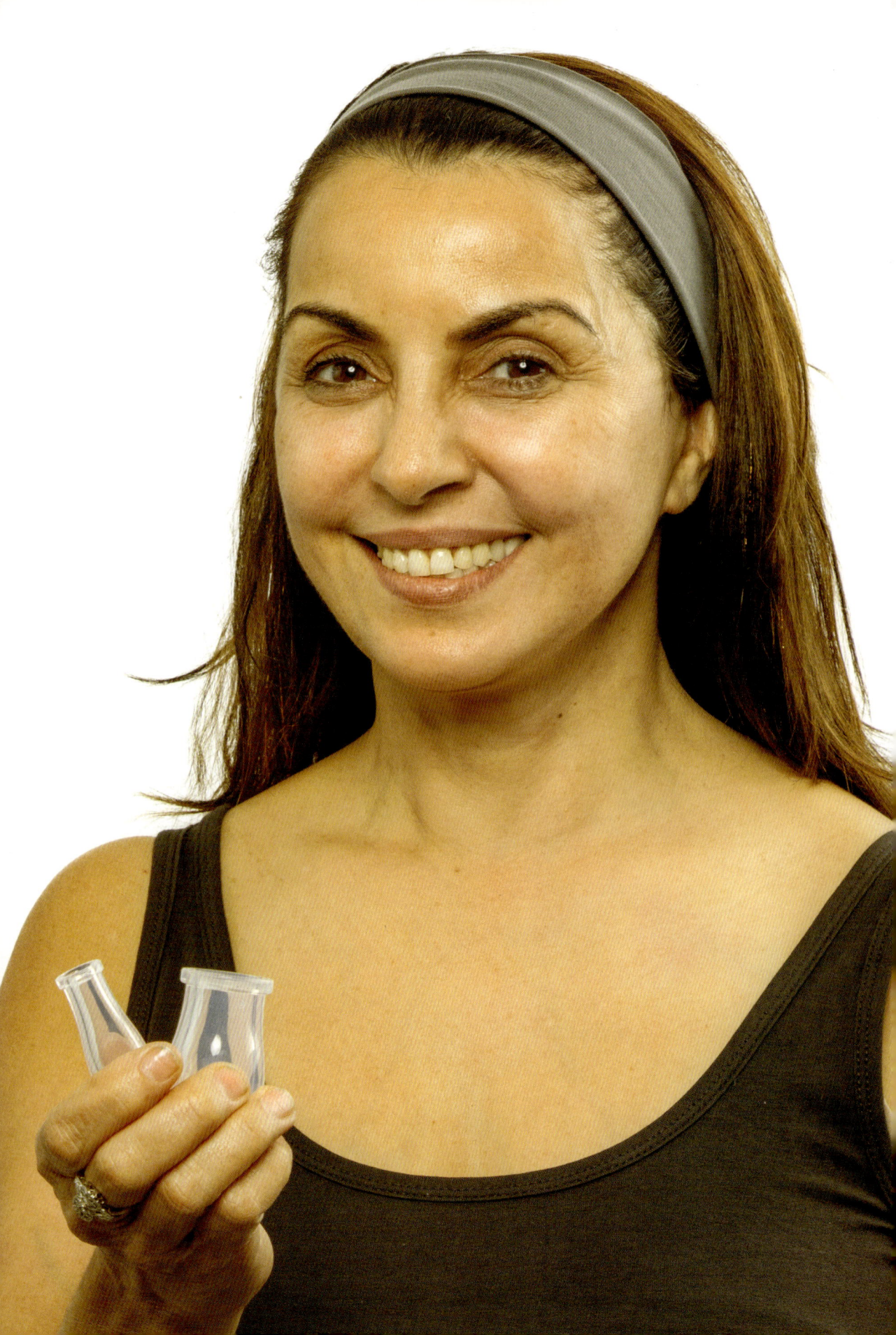

Overview of Treatment Process

A TOTAL FACE EXPERIENCE IN FIVE STEPS

WHAT DOES "a total face experience in five steps" mean? That means you need to begin with the neck and upper chest, then move on to the jawline, then the upper lip and cheek, then the forehead and finish with the delicate eye area. This sequence follows the natural lymphatic drainage patterns of the face and head.

Do not start or work on any region out of order, as this can have an adverse effect on the lymphatic activity in the face and head. Always follow the five steps laid out here in order.

> **BEFORE YOU BEGIN**
>
> *Remember to apply face oil before you start.* Be sure to apply a generous amount of face oil before you begin. You don't want to use so much oil that it is dripping, but use more than just a small amount. Don't forget to wipe your hands clean after you apply the oil and before you pick up the cup so it does not slip out of your hands.

WHERE TO BEGIN

WHEN WORKING ON both sides of the body, we generally work first on one side and then the other.

Practitioners usually follow general lymph drainage guidelines and begin with the left side of the body, which houses the more powerful drainage vessels. In clinical settings, there may be more advanced methods of bilateral application such as cupping machines.

In this book, we will always start on the left side of the face, address that side of the face entirely and then address the other.

> **LEFT SIDE FIRST**
> *Remember:* Treat the entire left side of your face before treating the right side of your face.

TREATMENT POINTERS

YOU MAY WANT to bookmark this page so you can be reminded of these points when you are treating yourself.

USE MOVING CUPS OR LIFT-AND-RELEASE TECHNIQUES — NO STATIONARY CUPS. Don't use stationary cups anywhere on the face or neck! Use lift-and-release, moving cups or the Morse Code of Cups combination of the two techniques to address every line of movement.

PRESSURE SHOULD BE LIGHT. If you want to keep the skin toned and tight and avoid cupping marks, the suction pressure must be light!

CUP SHOULD BE PROPORTIONAL TO THE FACE AND LARGER IN SIZE. Most face cupping sets have only a few sizes to choose from. Be sure to use the largest cup possible over any given area. See page 64.

THE APPLICATION SHOULD BE SLOW, RHYTHMIC AND REPETITIVE. Employ a slower pace, rhythmic movements and repetitive passes for the entire application. See page 62.

TREAT THE ENTIRE FACE EVENLY, ONE CUP-WIDTH AT A TIME. Also, to ensure an overall even treatment, repeat each pass three to five times.

> 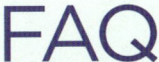 **CAN I FOCUS ON ONE AREA?**
>
> While you may want to focus on one area more than another, be sure to maintain this average number of passes across the entire face. If you really want, focus areas can receive two or three more passes than others, but do not overwork the area. Many passes can lead to swelling and cupping marks.

FOLLOW THE STEP-BY-STEP INSTRUCTIONS AS WRITTEN. It is important to follow the treatment steps as they are described and in the order in which they are written. The step-by-step instructions follow the natural lymph drainage process of the face and head.

LOOK FOR THE EXCEPTIONS. For each treatment, consider the "Exceptions and What-Ifs" notes in case you need to adjust the exact step-by-step process because of loose skin, facial hair, tight muscles or some other condition.

USE ONLY THE LIFT-AND-RELEASE TECHNIQUE IN THE FRONT OF THE NECK — NO MOVING CUPS. Remember the no-slide zone in the front of the neck! If you are unsure, do not use cups in the front of the neck. Instead, use your fingertips to do the cup-free options as suggested.

Understanding the Universal Pass

AS YOU BEGIN the facial cupping treatment process, it is important to become familiar with the front side of the neck, its delicate anatomy and the best method of application for treating this area. Considering how many nerves, blood vessels and lymph vessels are in this part of the neck, you must know a few safety points as you proceed.

You will begin your treatment with *Step 1: The Neck and Upper Chest*. The *Universal Pass*, which also focuses on this part of your body, is a procedure you will be repeating throughout your treatment.

WHY DO THE UNIVERSAL PASS?

STEP BY STEP, the cupping treatment in this book follows the general flow of lymph. (See pages 23–24 for more details on the lymphatic system.) Think of the Universal Pass as "unclogging a drain" so all the "garbage" — the lymph waste — can be thoroughly cleared from the region without obstruction.

When you do the Universal Pass, every section cleared in the face will then have a clear path for optimal lymph drainage. Some people can actually feel fluids collect and move through the front side of the neck during treatment. Others experience an increase in swallowing while working along this drainage route. These are welcome sensations of successful lymph drainage!

WHEN DO YOU DO THE UNIVERSAL PASS?

YOU'LL NOTICE that each step of the step-by-step treatment process in this book ends with the Universal Pass. The Universal Pass follows the exact same line of movement you will address in *Step 1: The Neck and Upper Chest*.

The route begins where your ear meets your jaw and travels diagonally down your neck to where the ultimate end point of all lymph drainage is, in your upper chest. For more details on how lymph drainage works, see pages 24 and 39.

This path travels over the big neck muscle called the sternocleidomastoid (SCM). To locate this muscle, simply turn your head to the side then bend it forward slightly; the SCM muscle will "pop" forward for you to identify it.

Then, when you get down to the center of the upper chest where the collarbones are, the path bends under the collarbones and around to upper chest points. When you look at the instructional image, imagine this line of movement as a diagonal *L* for moving *Lymph* fluid.

> **DID YOU KNOW?**
> Cupping along the SCM muscle not only stimulates all the lymph drainage; it also offers great relief to neck and jaw tension, too.

In *Step 1*, you will treat the front side of your neck many times to stimulate the lymphatic activity in your neck and upper chest before you begin the entire treatment process. After every step of the process, as each section of the face is cleared, you will find instructions to repeat the Universal Pass. You want to keep the lymph "garbage" moving along its disposal route.

Be sure that you are comfortable with the process, and follow the rules of application every time.

RULES OF APPLICATION FOR THE UNIVERSAL PASS

USE ONLY LIFT-AND RELEASE IN THE FRONT OF YOUR NECK. The blood and lymph capillaries that attach just under the skin will be safely stimulated and the nerves will not be irritated. No stationary cups here. No moving cups either. This region is designated a no-slide zone for safety and optimal effectiveness.

PROGRESS IN A DOWNWARD DIRECTION ONLY. As you work, always proceed from the face downward. Move diagonally down the neck and toward the upper chest. If you work in an upward direction, you will incorrectly influence the regional lymph fluids, which can potentially lead to head congestion or an overload of the lymph nodes.

IF YOU COME ACROSS ANY VISIBLE BLOOD VESSELS, TRY TO SKIP OVER THAT AREA ENTIRELY. If you happen to attach a cup over these vital blood vessels, however, especially those that pulse, it should be fine. Just be sure to follow the rules: lift-and-release only in this region. But try to avoid visible blood vessels in the first place.

USE SLOW, RHYTHMIC AND REPETITIVE MOVEMENTS. It is especially important to work mindfully in the front of your neck. Not only is this region hypersensitive, but the vagus nerve travels through the front of the neck. Any erratic, vigorous or aggressive applications in this region could irritate the vagus nerve and cause nausea, dizziness or headaches.

THE UNIVERSAL PASS: KEEP IT SIMPLE!

DON'T OVERTHINK IT. The most important thing to remember is that the neck is a no-slide zone. Lift-and-release only, progressing downward along that *L* line of movement.

DON'T SKIP IT. No matter which method you choose, with a cup or without, be sure not to skip over the Universal Pass. Your treatment will not be as successful if you avoid the front of the neck entirely.

SAFETY FIRST: Never use stationary cups, moving cups, strong suction or vigorous movements in the front of your neck. Use only lift-and-release. Just follow the rules of the Universal Pass!

UNIVERSAL PASS ICON

This icon will appear at the end of each step as a reminder to complete the Universal Pass after completing the treatment.

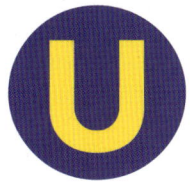

THE UNIVERSAL PASS

LOCATION
This area includes the jump-off location under the earlobe, the front of the neck over the SCM muscle, and the upper chest, just under the collarbone. This is the same location as for *Step 1*.

STARTING POINT
Start in the soft space of your neck, just under the jump-off location from your face where the jaw meets the earlobe. (See the star in the photo.)

LINE OF MOVEMENT
Follow along down the diagonal *L* line from the starting point, along the SCM muscle, ending at the upper chest locations. (See the Xs.) Picture this line of movement as a diagonal *L* for moving *Lymph*.

END POINT
End at the upper chest, the same location addressed in *Step 1*. The Universal Pass follows the same exact line of movement as in *Step 1*.

TREATMENT PROCESS
- Squeeze the cup, then gently attach it at the starting point.

- Simply lift the skin with a little suction, then squeeze the cup again to detach it from the skin's surface. That's the lift-and-release technique!

- Repeat this lift-and-release process four or five times down that diagonal line (the Xs) toward the end point in the upper chest.

- Once you finish that diagonal *L* line of movement, that's it! This will be the line of movement for every Universal Pass mentioned in each step of your treatment process.

> The *jump-off location* is where the jawline meets the earlobe on the face. This location will be identified again in *Step 2* when you are treating the jawline.

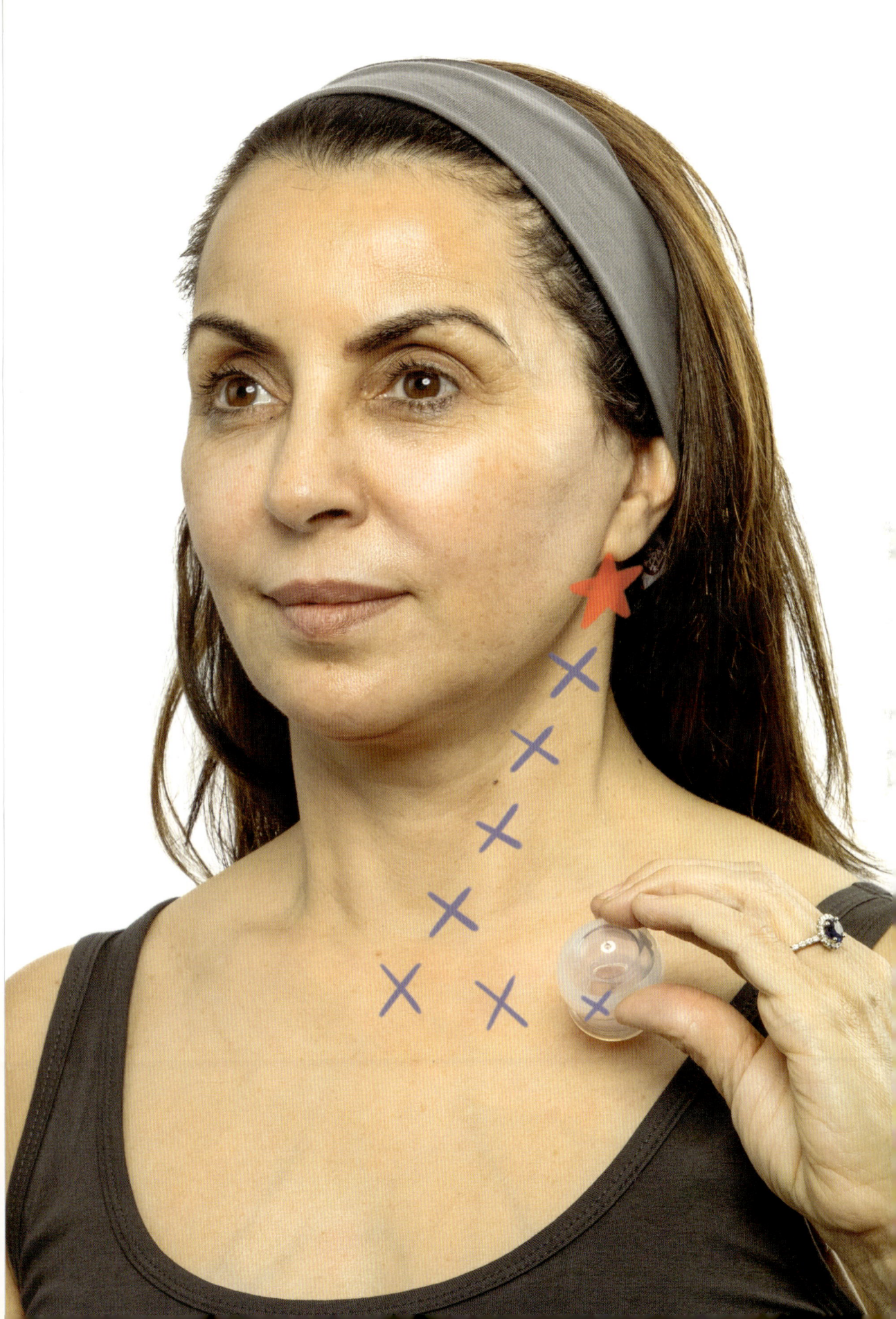

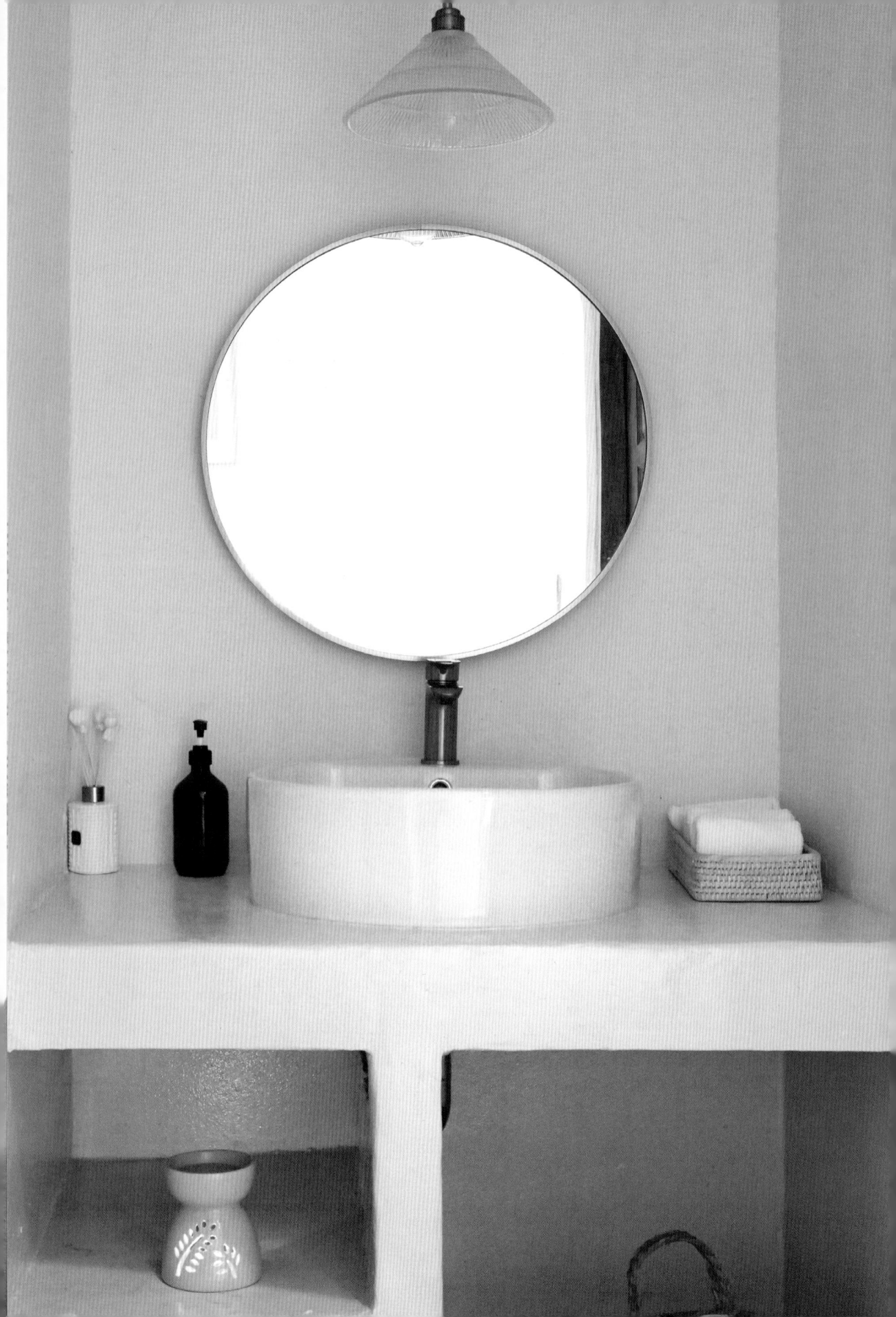

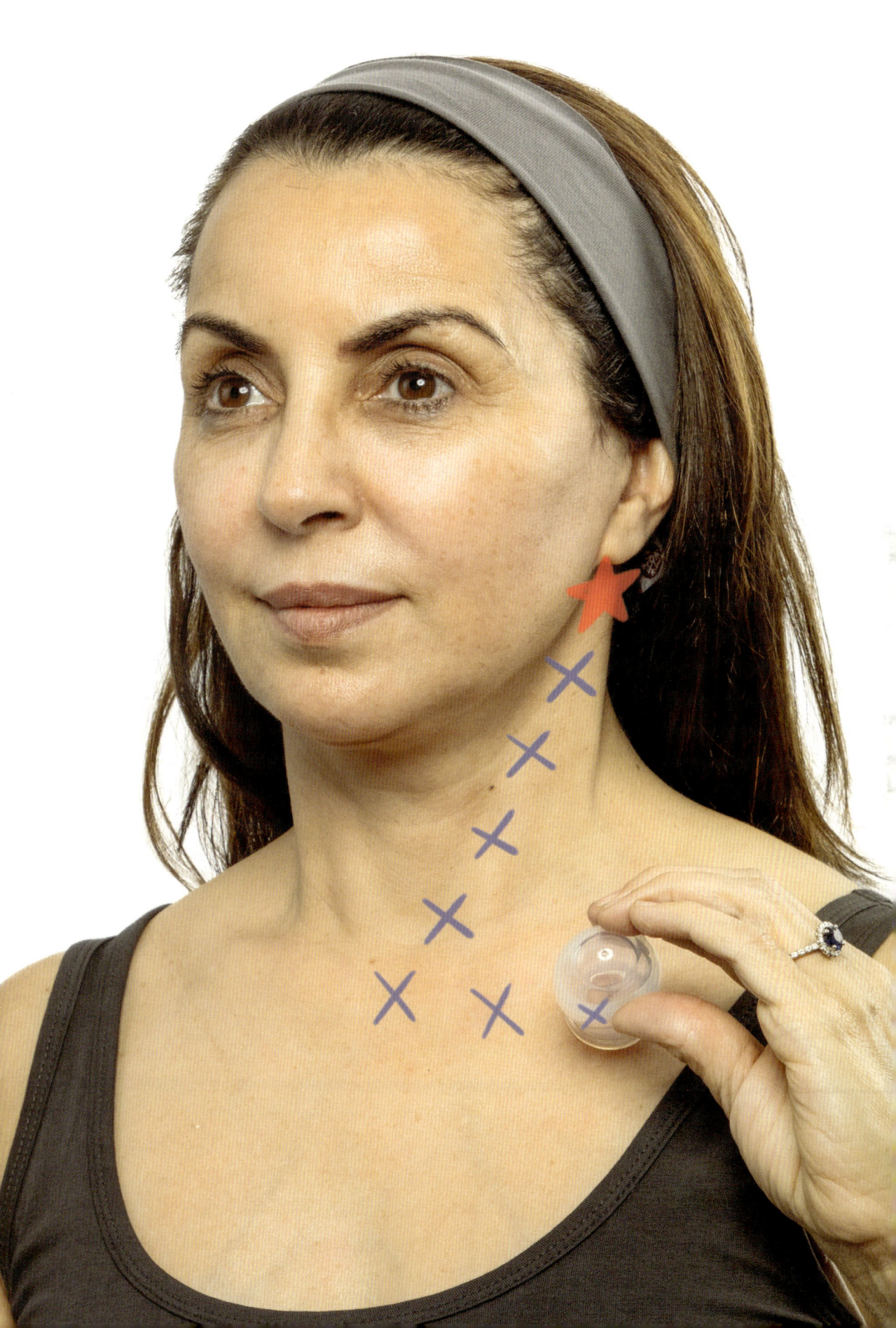

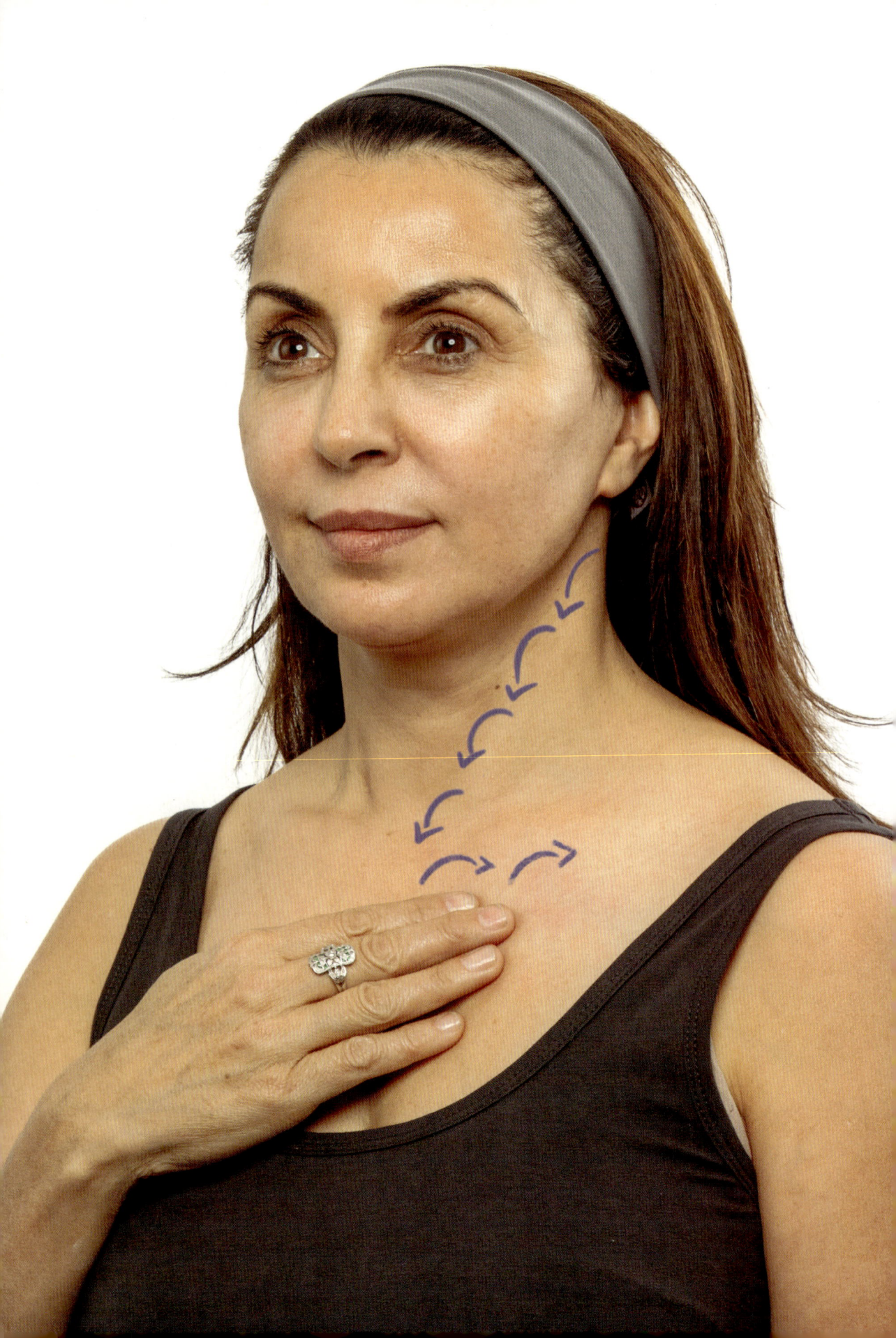

THE UNIVERSAL PASS

Cup-Free Option

WHILE CUPPING along the front of the neck may seem intimidating, it's not. Every person I have taught how to do this has had immediate success and positive results, as long as they followed the rules.

If you are unsure about using a cup in this delicate region, simply put the cup down and use the cup-free option shown. It is simple, safe and incredibly effective.

TREATMENT PROCESS

- Use the same starting point, line of movement and end point as instructed with cups, but with your fingertips. Your intention here is only to stretch the skin, to stimulate the underlying lymph capillaries for lymph drainage, so be sure to keep the pressure very light.

- For this cup-free option, reach across the front of your neck. When working on the left side of the face, use your right hand instead of your left; similarly, use your left hand on the right side of your face. See the photo.

- Starting at the top of your neck, where the jaw meets the ear, gently use your flattened fingers to contact the skin's surface. Make a half-circle, slightly stretching the skin up, forward and down, like the arc of a rainbow.

- Repeat this gentle skin-stretching, half-circle method of application one hand-width at a time and make your way down to the top of the upper chest area end points. The average neck will accommodate three hand-widths, but everybody is different; what's most important is to address the entire region.

- You can use this cup-free method of application any time the Universal Pass is called for in your treatment process.

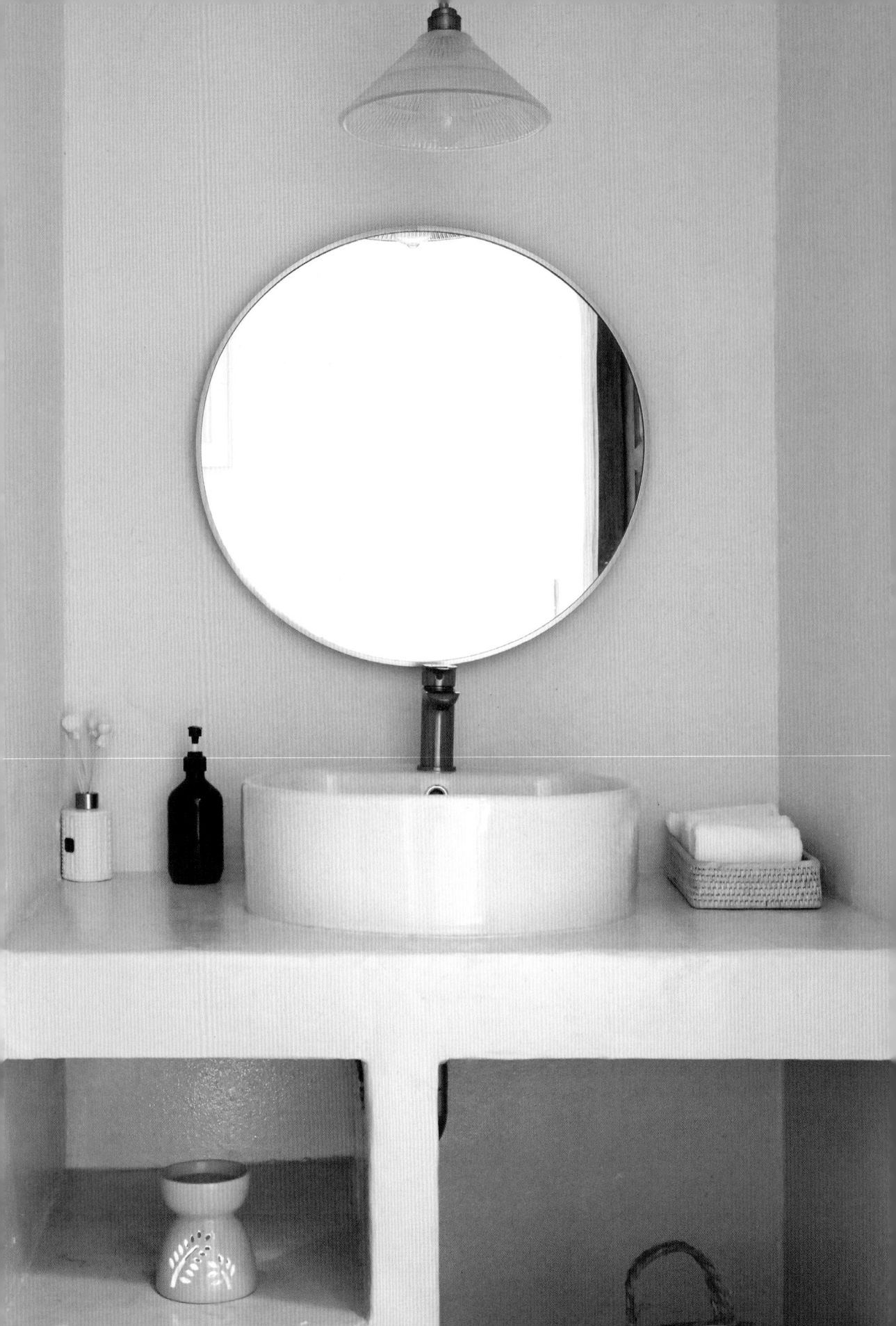

FOLLOW THE STEP-BY-STEP INSTRUCTIONS WITH THE FACE-CUPPING MAP

The following step-by-step instructions are meant to be followed alongside the *Face-Cupping Map* (page 150). I recommend you read each step first and review it as needed alongside the *Face-Cupping Map* as you work in front of a mirror.

To complete the treatment, simply follow the numbered sections, treat each section of the face evenly (using the same number of passes over every cup-width), repeat the Universal Pass where indicated and then continue to the next section. There are five steps in all.

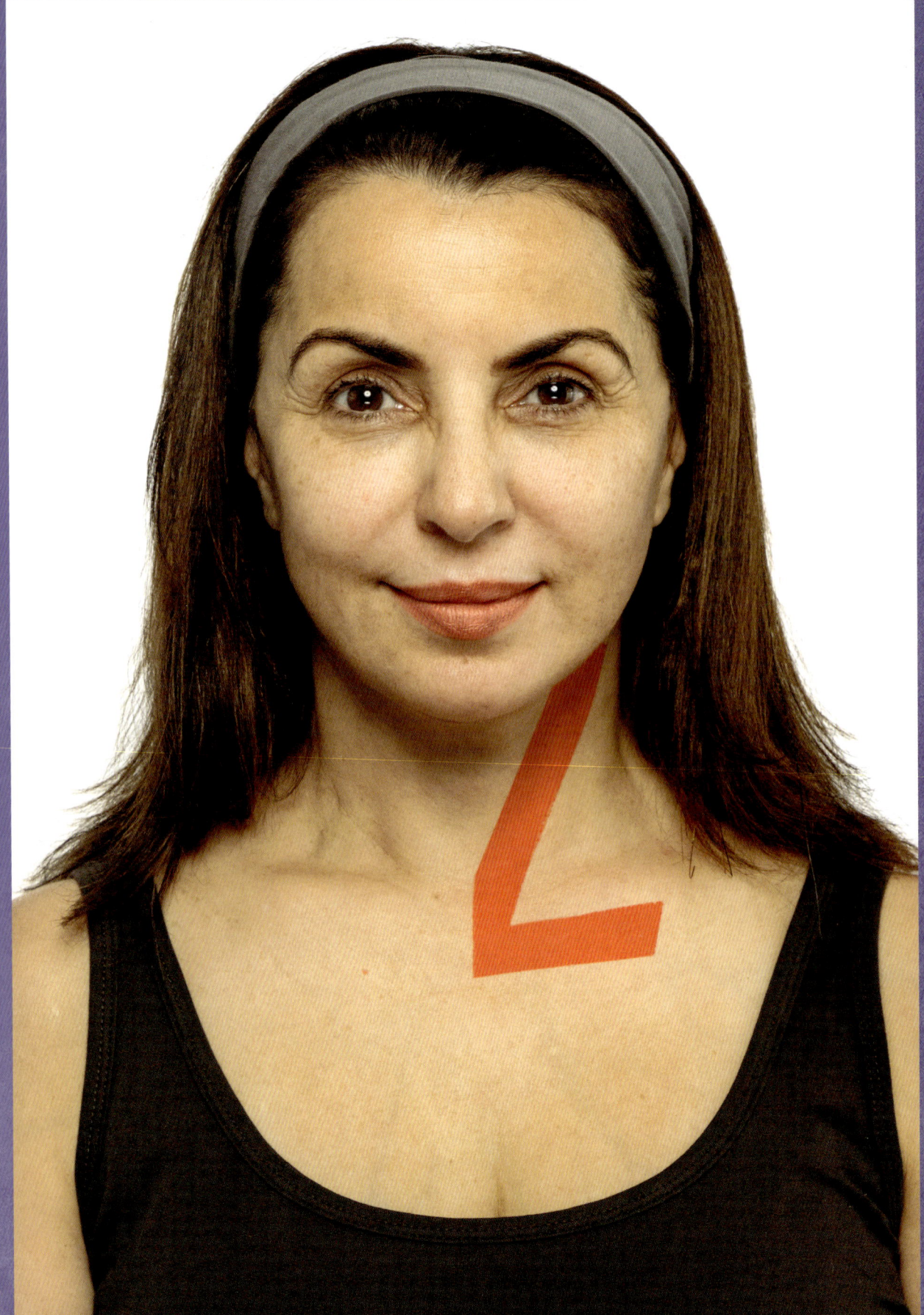

STEP 1
THE NECK AND UPPER CHEST

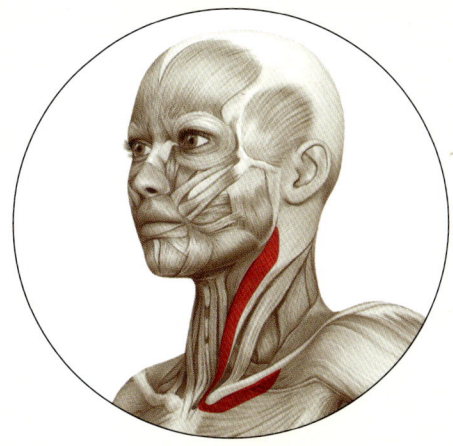

WHY CUP YOUR NECK AND UPPER CHEST?

THIS IS THE BEST PLACE to begin your treatment. It is important to address the upper chest and neck regions before addressing the face, since this begins the lymphatic drainage process for the entire head. Starting here will "unclog the drain" for lymphatic movement, so everything you drain from the face will efficiently drain into the thoracic ducts in the upper chest.

Remember, this is the exact same line of movement as for the Universal Pass, which you will repeat after each of the five treatment steps.

Additionally, this line of movement travels directly over a very tight neck muscle, your sternocleidomastoid or SCM muscle, so any neck tension you are feeling when you start the treatment will relax with every cupping pass.

> **HOW MANY PASSES?**
> The many passes in *Step 1: The Neck and Upper Chest* are necessary to stimulate lymph drainage for the entire face and head. *Step 1* is the only time you will need to complete as many passes for this line of movement. When doing the Universal Pass after each section is cleared, you need to do it only one to three times.

THE NECK AND UPPER CHEST

LOCATION
This area includes the jump-off location under the earlobe, the front of the neck over the SCM muscle, and the upper chest, just under the collarbone. This is the same location for the Universal Pass.

STARTING POINT
Start in the soft space of your neck, just below the jump-off location where the jaw meets the earlobe. (See the star in the photo.)

LINE OF MOVEMENT
Follow along down the diagonal *L* line from the starting point, along the SCM muscle, ending at the upper chest locations. (See the Xs.) Picture this line of movement as a diagonal *L* for moving *Lymph*.

END POINT
End at the upper chest, in the soft space just below the collarbone. (See the blue X in the photo.)

> *Remember:* The location, starting point, line of movement and end point are the same for *Step 1: The Neck and Upper Chest* and for the Universal Pass.

TREATMENT PROCESS
- Squeeze the cup, then gently attach it at the starting point.
- Using lift-and-release only, follow the line of movement down the side of the neck, along the SCM muscle and into those upper chest locations.
- A shorter neck may require three or four cup placements to accomplish this, a longer neck may require five or six cup placements.
- Repeat this lift-and-release process along the line of movement six to nine times. Continue to *Step 2: The Jawline*.

> *Caution:* This region involves the anterior triangle endangerment sites, so it's lift-and-release only.

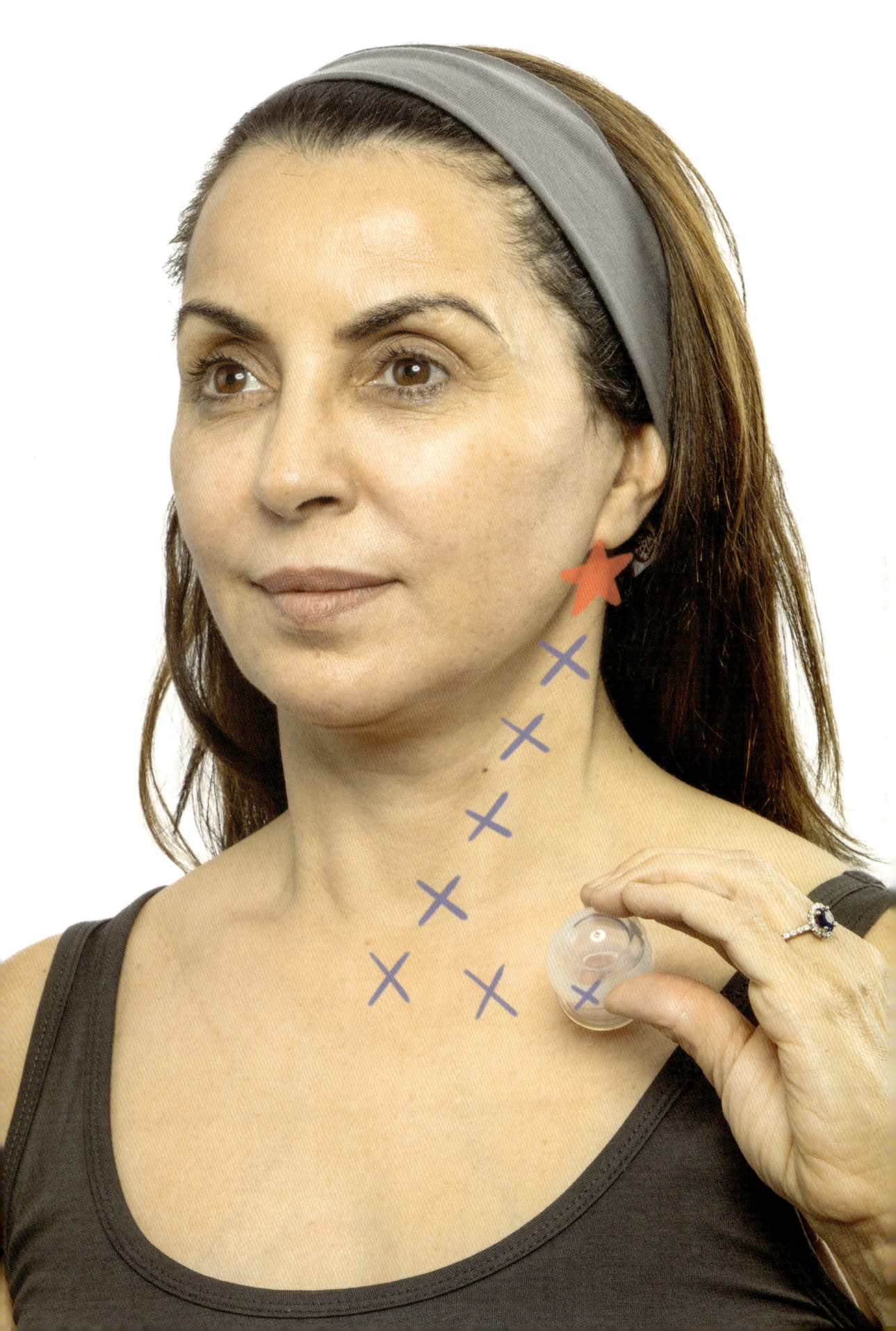

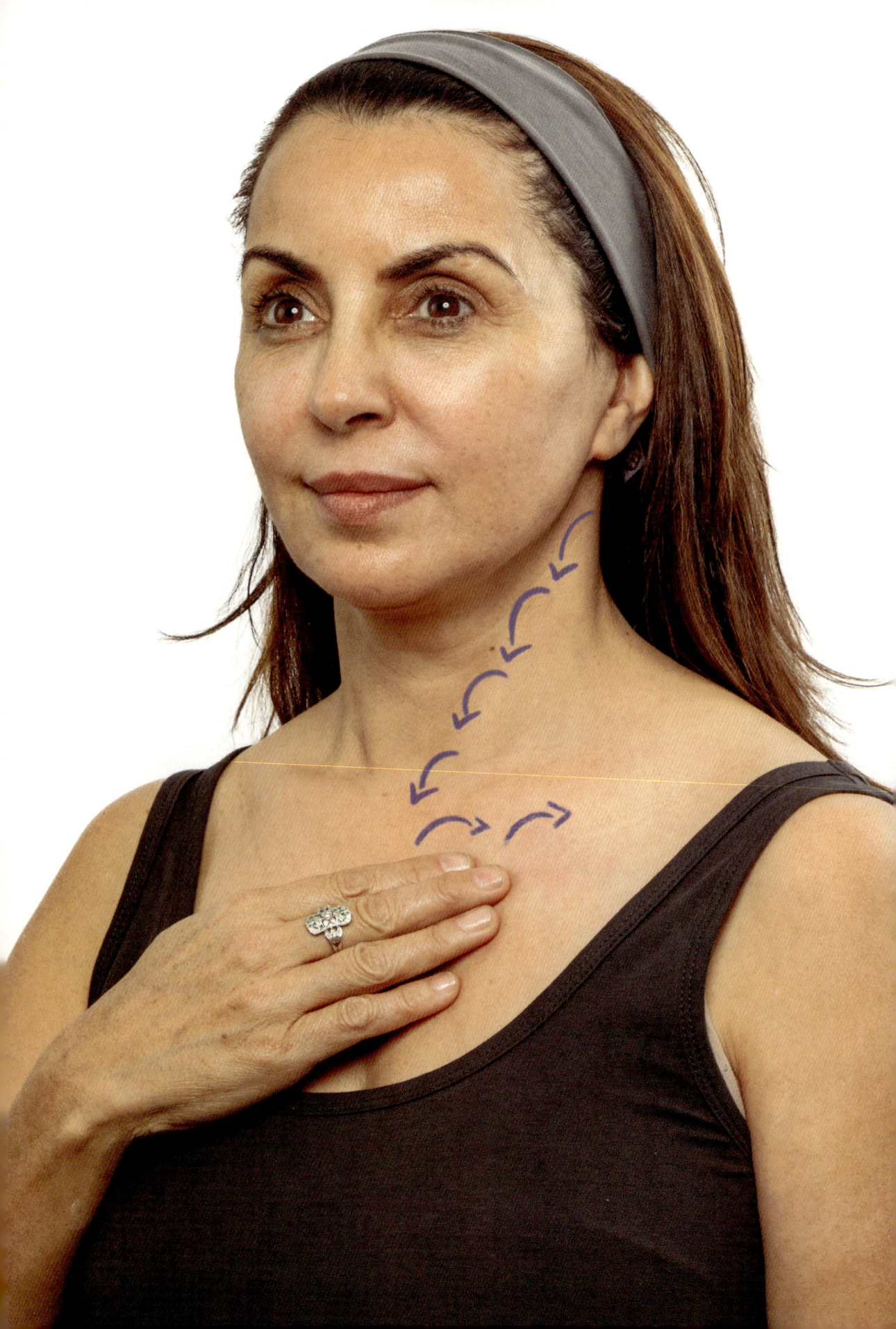

THE NECK AND UPPER CHEST

Cup-Free Option

If a cup will not attach to your skin in this section for any reason (for example, facial hair), or if you prefer to be cautious using a cup in this area, simply use your fingertips to gently follow the lymph drainage pathways.

TREATMENT PROCESS
Use the opposite hand of the side of the neck you are addressing to reach across the front of your neck for this cup-free option. If working on the left side of the face, use your right hand, and vice versa. See the photo.

- Starting at the top of neck where the jaw meets the ear, gently use your flattened fingers to contact the skin's surface and make a half-circle, slightly stretching the skin up, forward and down (see photo), like an arc of a rainbow.

- Repeat this gentle skin-stretching, half-circle method of application one hand-width at a time and make your way down to the top of the upper chest area end points. The average neck will accommodate three hand-widths, but everybody is different; what's most important is to address the entire region.

- Repeat this cup-free method of application for every time the Universal Pass is mentioned hereafter.

- *Keep it light:* Remember the intention here is to stretch the skin only, as we are attempting to stimulate the underlying lymph capillaries for lymph drainage, so be sure to keep the pressure light.

> **EXCEPTIONS AND WHAT-IFS**
> **FACIAL HAIR?** Follow these cup-free recommendations.

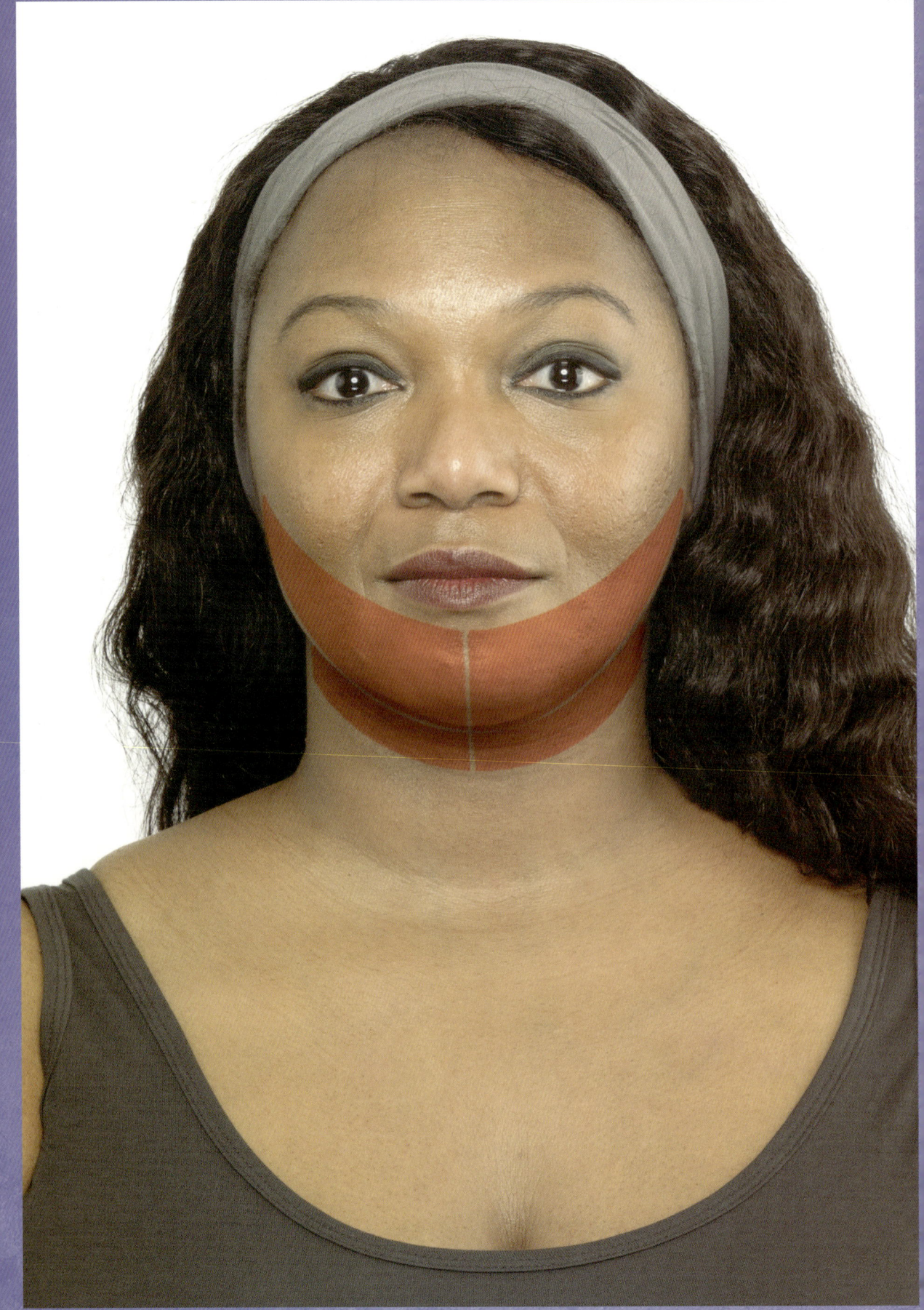

STEP 2
THE JAWLINE

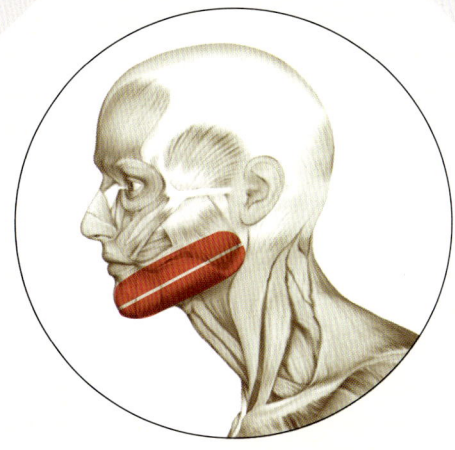

WHY CUP YOUR JAWLINE?

YOUR JAWLINE may be the first location where you notice your skin beginning to sag. You may even notice those concentrated areas of loose skin we know as jowls.

Or you may suffer from pain and tightness in your jaw and neck. The jawline area has many blood vessels, lymph nodes and muscles, so any tension there can contribute to pains in the jaw and neck. This tension can also inhibit circulation to the skin.

> **LYMPHATICS FYI**
> You may be familiar with the lymphatic activity here, as several lymph nodes along the underside of the jawline are the first to swell when you have head congestion or at the onset of a cold or flu-like illness.

Cupping can stimulate microcirculation in the area being cupped, which helps to improve your complexion, tonicity, overall appearance and general health of the tissue. Additionally, cupping can release muscle tension along your jawline, offering relief to jaw and neck muscles.

For the greatest benefits, we divide the cupping treatment into two parts: below the jawline and above the jawline. Note that there are also cup-free options for both parts.

BELOW THE JAWLINE

LOCATION
This area is along the underside of the face and jawbone, not across the front of the neck, which is an endangerment site (see page 68).

STARTING POINT
Start in the center of the jawline, under the chin.

LINE OF MOVEMENT
Follow along the underside of the entire jawbone.

END POINT
End in front of the ear and under the contour of your jawbone where the jaw meets the ear. (See cup location in photo.) This is just below the jump-off location, where the Universal Pass begins.

TREATMENT PROCESS
- Attach the cup at the starting point and follow the line of movement using lift-and-release and/or moving cups to the end point.
- Repeat this movement three to five times.
- Repeat the Universal Pass one to three times before proceeding.
- Continue to the next part, *Above the Jawline*.

> **EXCEPTIONS AND WHAT-IFS**
>
> **VERY LOOSE SKIN?** Use the lift-and-release technique; as the skin tones up, add in moving cups if desired.
>
> **JAW TENSION?** Do not force the cup to move across an area of resistance. Finish the line of movement with lift-and-release, moving cups or the Morse Code of Cups technique.
>
> **FACIAL HAIR?** Follow the cup-free recommendations.

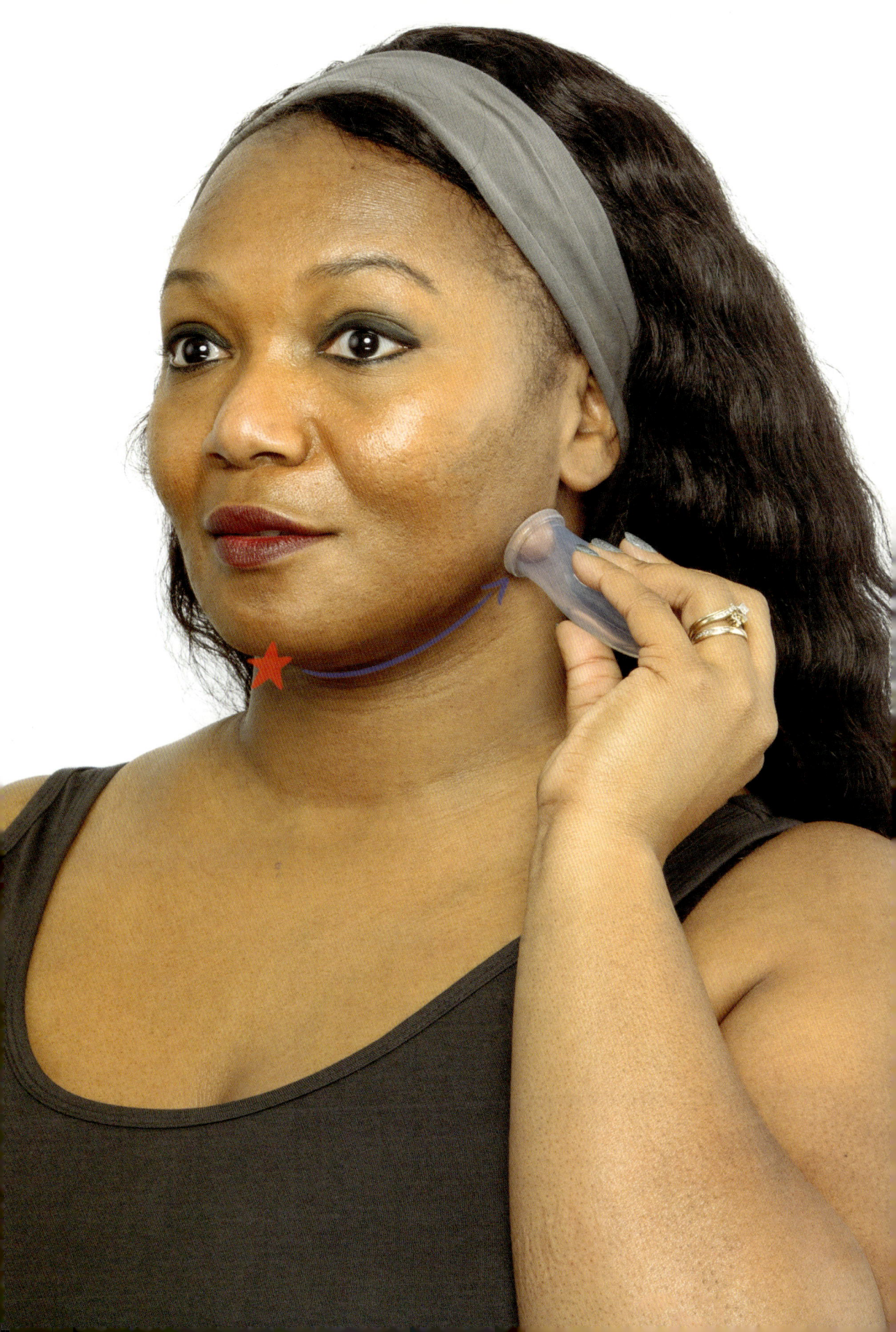

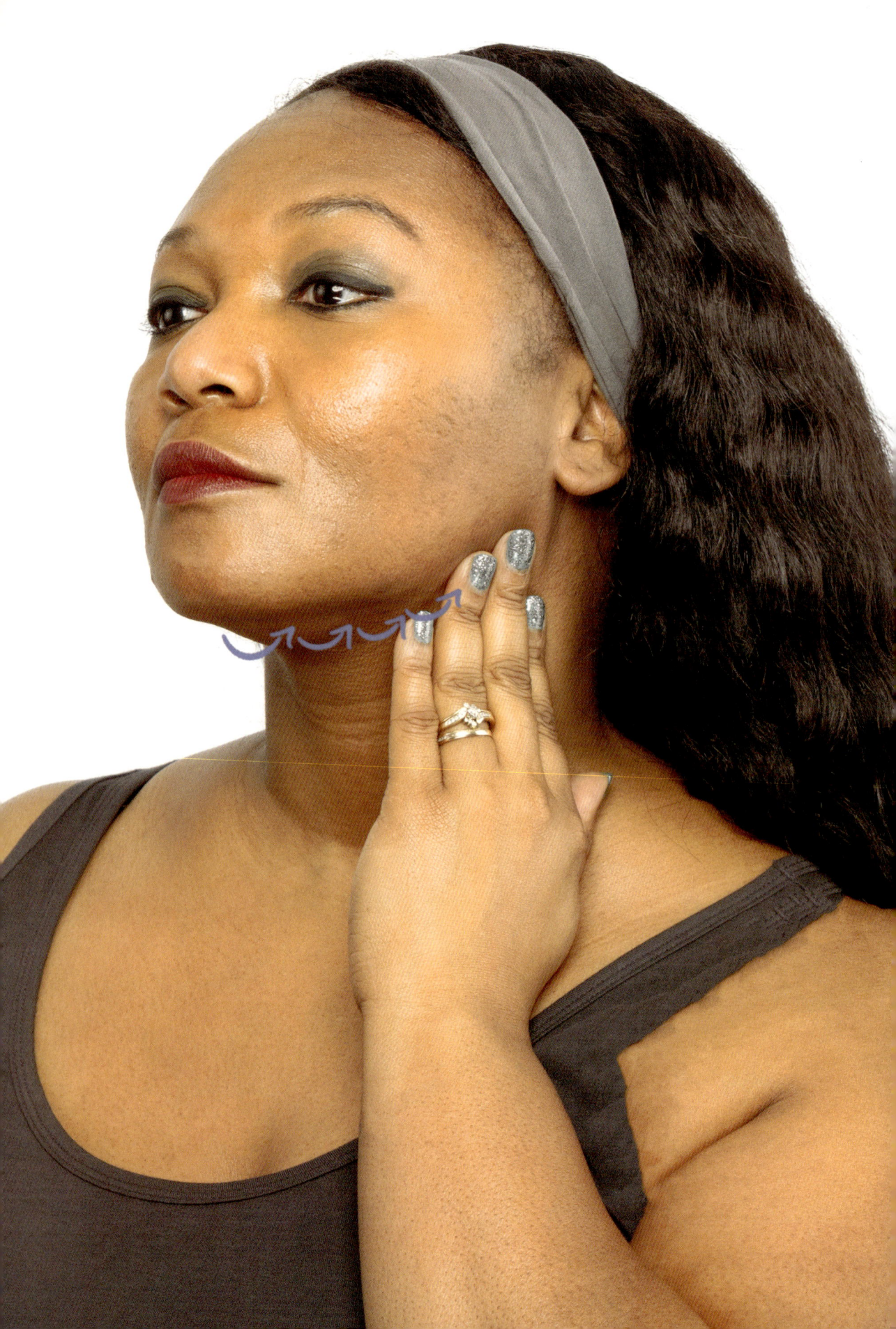

BELOW THE JAWLINE

Cup-Free Option

If the cups will not work in this region for whatever reason (facial hair, cosmetic implants, etc.), simply use your fingertips to gently follow the lymph drainage pathways.

TREATMENT PROCESS
Using the same starting point, line of movement and end point as instructed with cups, use your fingertips to create small half-circles across the surface of your skin.

- Begin your fingertip half-circles in the center of your jawline, under your chin.

- As you treat the left side of your face, your fingertips will lightly stretch the skin slightly downward and around toward the left ear. When treating the right side, your fingertips will move down and around toward your right ear.

- Completely remove your fingertips from your skin after every half-circle is completed, then "step" your fingertips to the next starting place and repeat. Do this until you have covered the entire line of movement.

- Repeat the Universal Pass one to three times before proceeding to the next step, *Above the Jawline*.

While every face is different, you will probably do four or five half-circles on each side of your face. Remember, you are only trying to stimulate the lymph capillaries, so the pressure should remain very light.

ABOVE THE JAWLINE

LOCATION
This area is below the mouth and along the jawline and ends in front of the earlobe. Be sure to not pull any lip tissue into the cup, as that is not part of this section.

STARTING POINT
In the center of the chin, under the lower lip.

LINE OF MOVEMENT
Follow along the entire jawbone, progressing toward the ears.

END POINT
End in front of the ear on the face, where the jawbone meets the ear. (See cup location in photo). This is also the jump-off location, where the Universal Pass begins.

TREATMENT PROCESS
- Attach the cup at the starting point.
- Follow the line of movement using lift-and-release and/or moving cups to the end point.
- Repeat this movement three to five times.
- Repeat the Universal Pass one to three times before proceeding.
- Continue to *Step 3: The Cheeks and Upper Lip*.

> **EXCEPTIONS AND WHAT-IFS**
> See the recommendations on page 82 for dealing with very loose skin, jaw tension or facial hair along the jawline.

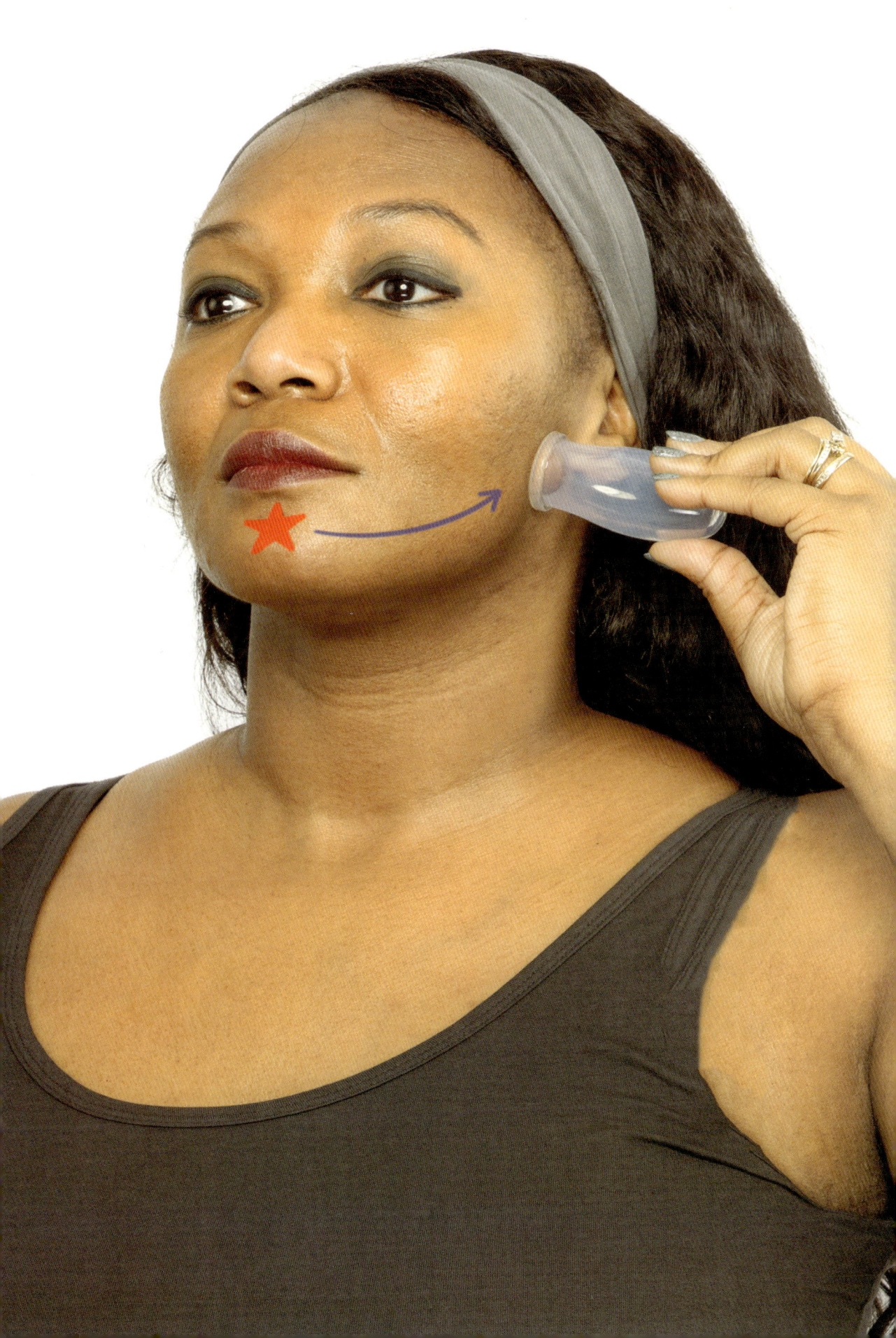

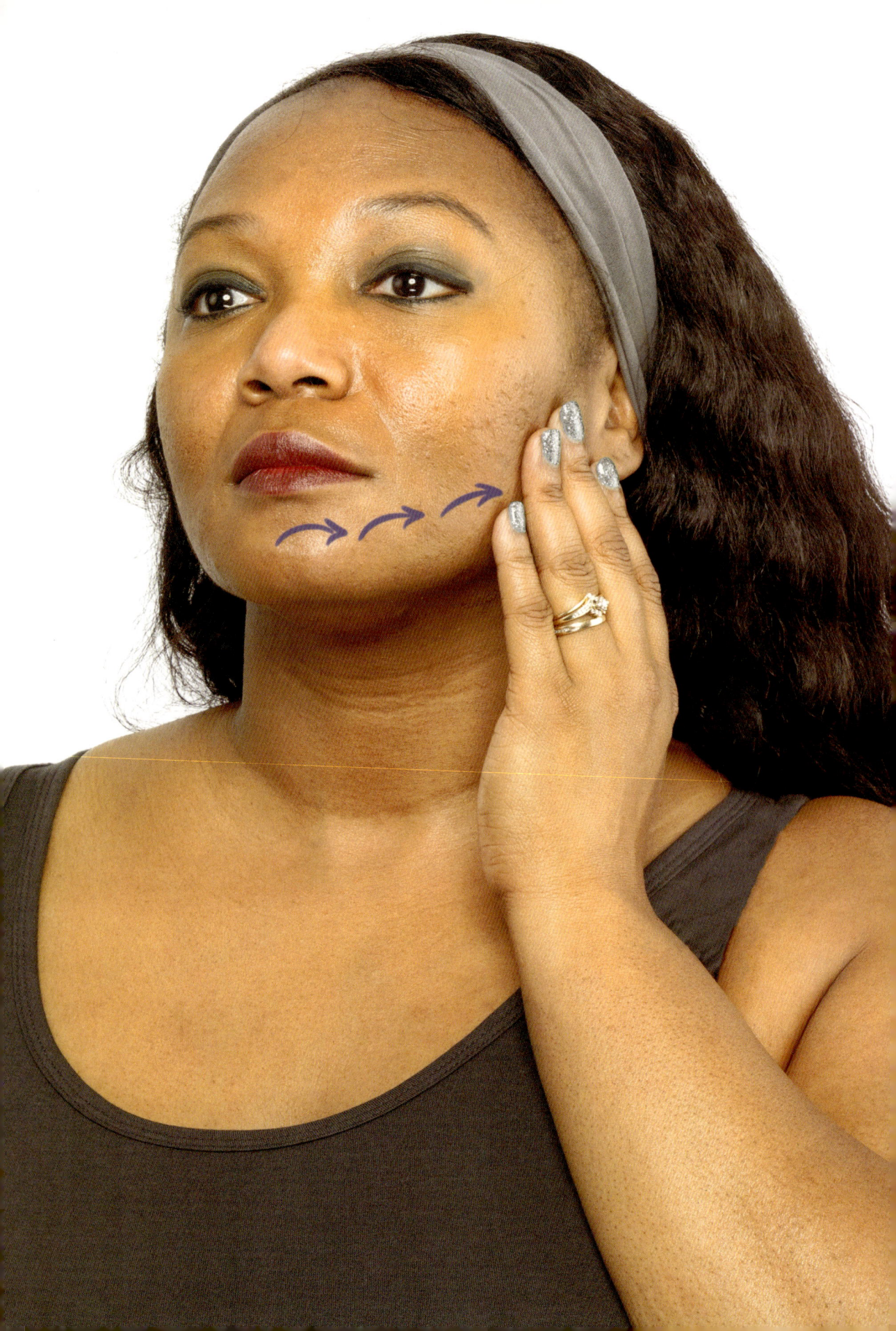

ABOVE THE JAWLINE

Cup-Free Option

If the cups will not work for whatever reason in this region (facial hair, cosmetic implants, etc.), simply use your fingertips to gently follow the lymph drainage pathways.

TREATMENT PROCESS

Using the same starting point, line of movement and end point as instructed with cups, use your fingertips to create small half-circles across the surface of the skin.

- Begin your fingertip half-circles at your chin.

- As you treat the left side of your face, your fingertips will lightly stretch the skin slightly upward and around toward the left ear. When treating the right side, your fingertips will move upward and around toward your right ear.

- Completely remove your fingertips from your skin after every half-circle is completed, then "step" your fingertips to the next starting place and repeat. Do this until you have covered the entire line of movement.

- Repeat the Universal Pass one to three times before proceeding to *Step 3: The Cheeks and Upper Lip*.

- While every face is different, you will probably complete four or five half-circles on each side of your face. Remember, you are only trying to stimulate the lymph capillaries, so the pressure should remain very light.

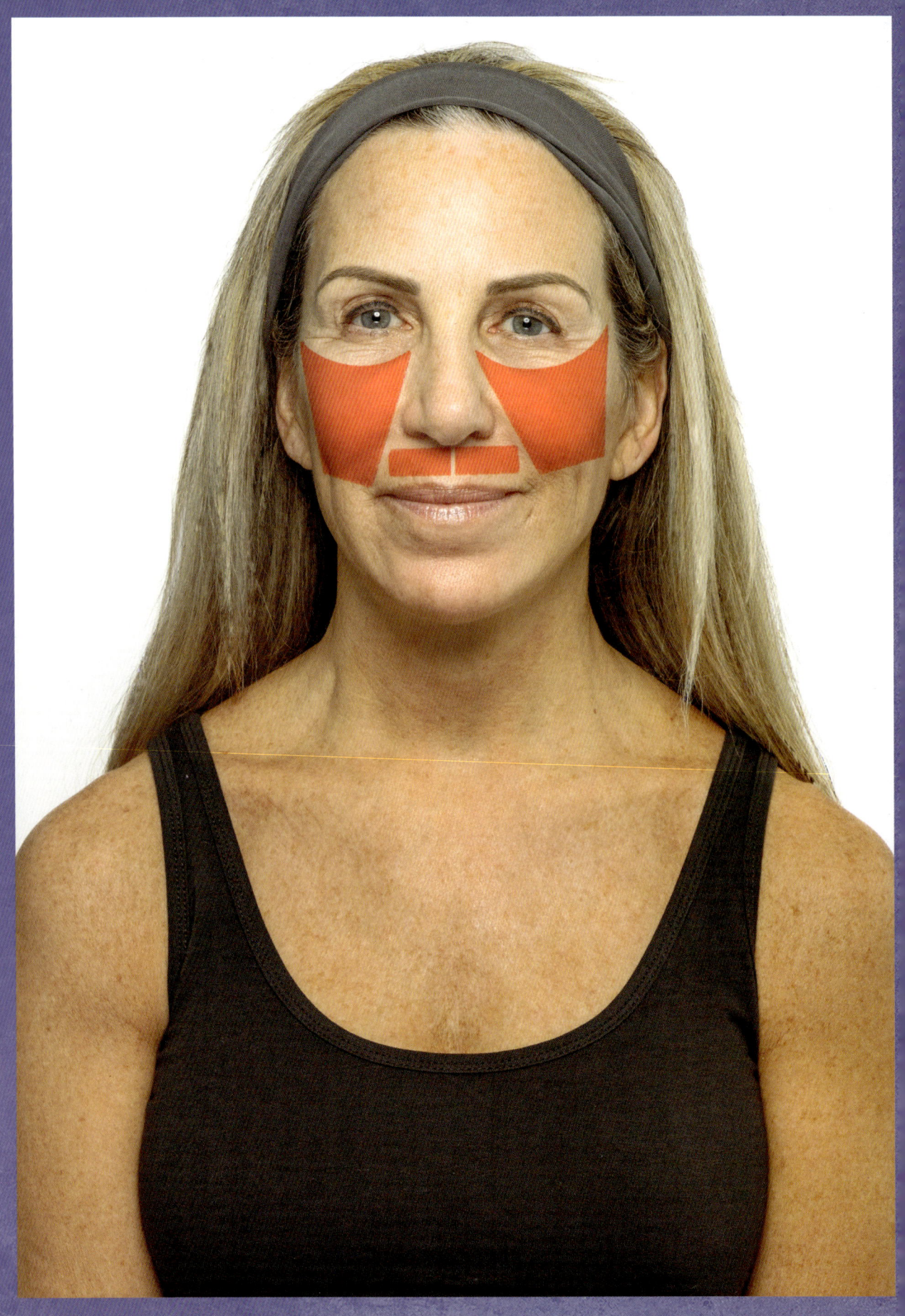

STEP 3
THE CHEEKS AND UPPER LIP

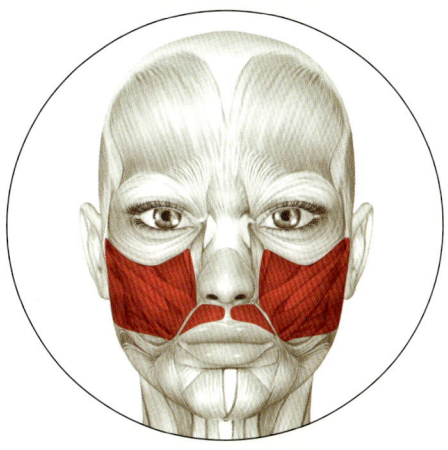

WHY CUP YOUR CHEEKS AND UPPER LIP?

YOUR CHEEKS cover a large surface of your face and they showcase much of your facial skin's health. Your skin can sag here, too, and the jaw muscles in this area can contribute to muscle tension. Also, the connection between your cheek and upper lip can contribute to "smile lines" at the corners of your mouth as well as other wrinkles across the upper lip area.

Cupping stimulates microcirculation, which will bring a healthy glow across the cheeks. Wrinkles will soften and muscle tension will ease when you cup this entire cheek and upper lip region.

For the greatest benefits, we divide the cupping treatment into two parts: the upper lip and the cheeks. The upper lip is a very small area, so it is addressed quickly before the entire cheek. Note that there are also cup-free options for both parts.

> **CUP CHOICE**
> For the upper lip, you will need a small cup. For the cheek, you will need a larger cup.

THE UPPER LIP

LOCATION
This is a very small area above the mouth; the cup should not enter the nostril or pull any lip tissue into the cup.

STARTING POINT
Start in the center of the upper lip, below the nose and above the lip.

LINE OF MOVEMENT
Move from the center of the upper lip to just above the corner of the mouth, where the cheek begins.

END POINT
End above the corner of the mouth and below the nostril. The upper lip section generally ends where your smile line wrinkles are. (This is where you will begin treating the cheek.)

TREATMENT PROCESS
Be sure to use a smaller cup to treat the upper lip.

- Attach cup at the starting point and follow the line of movement using lift-and-release and/or moving cups to the end point.

- Repeat this movement three to five times.

- You don't need to do the Universal Pass after you finish treating your upper lip. Simply continue to the next part of *Step 3, The Cheeks*.

> **EXCEPTIONS AND WHAT-IFS**
>
> **FACIAL HAIR?** Follow the cup-free recommendations.
>
> **RECENT COSMETIC INJECTIONS?** Don't treat until 30 days post-injection. When you do treat, use lift-and-release or, the closer you are to the procedure, follow the cup-free recommendations.

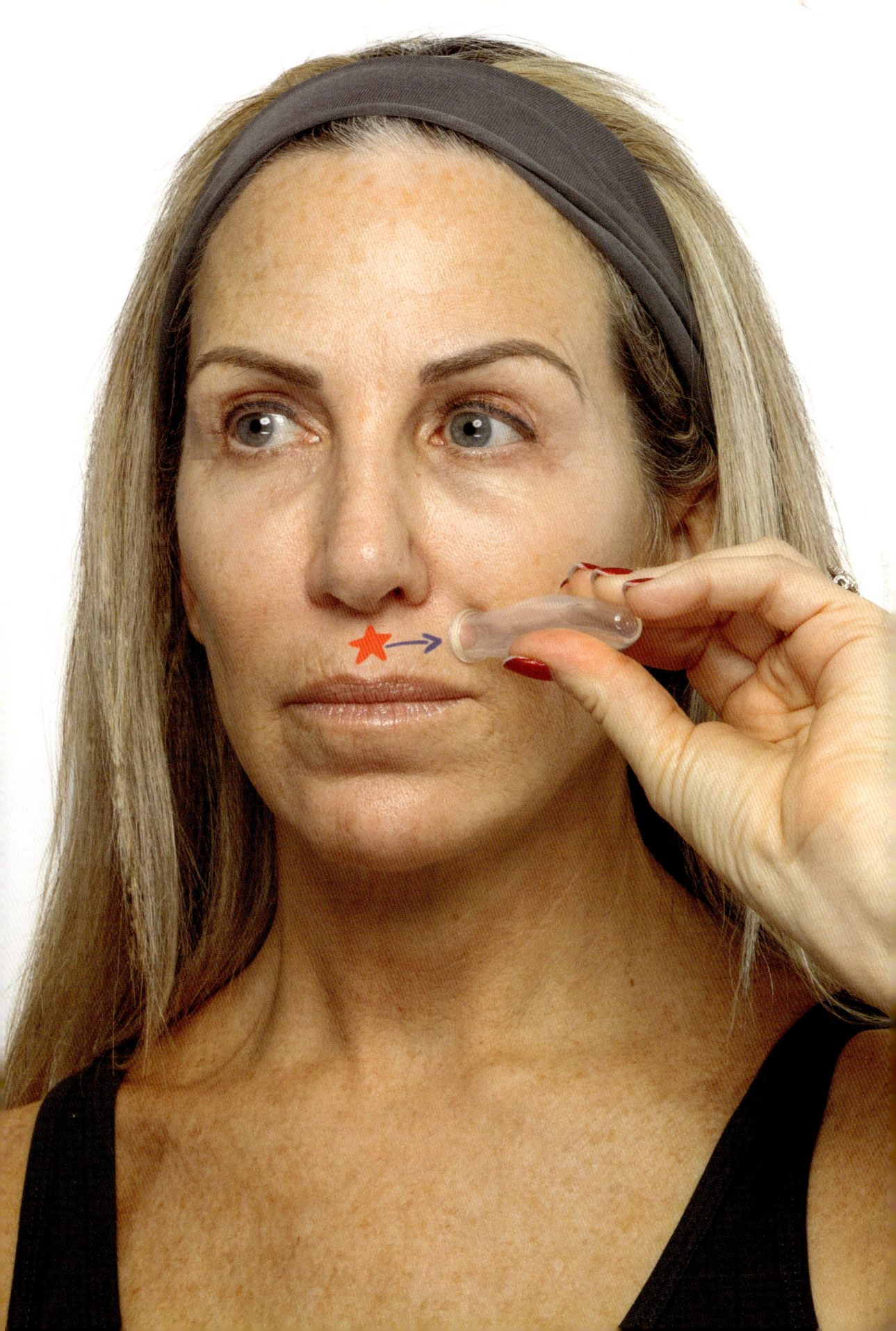

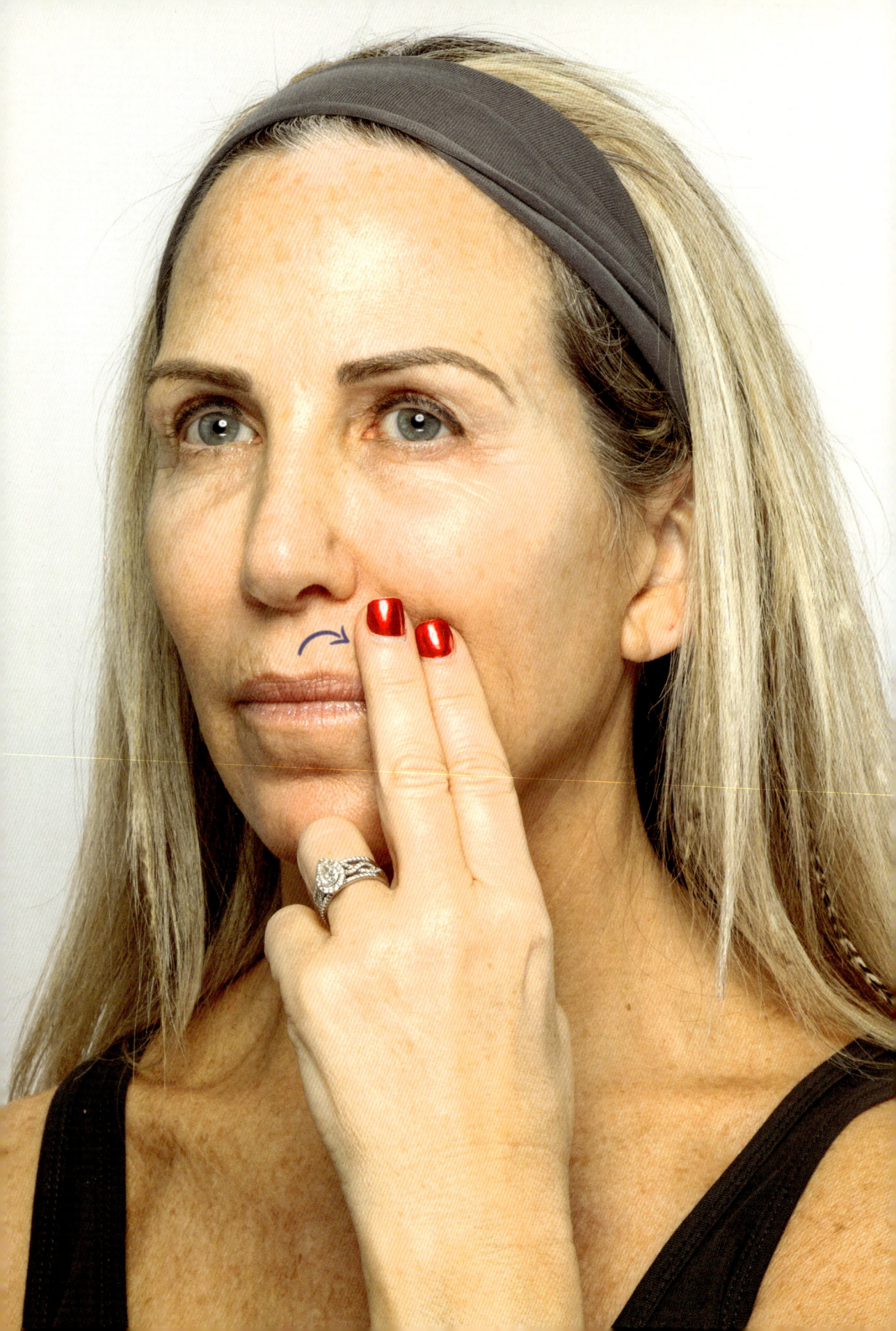

THE UPPER LIP

Cup-Free Option

If the cups will not work in this region for whatever reason (facial hair, cosmetic injections, etc.), simply use your fingertips to gently follow the lymph drainage pathways.

TREATMENT PROCESS
Using the same starting point, line of movement and end point as instructed with cups, use your fingertips to create small half-circles across the surface of your skin.

- Begin your fingertip half-circles in the center of your upper lip, under the center of your nostrils.

- As you treat the left side of your face, your fingertips will lightly stretch the skin slightly upward and around toward the left side of your mouth. When treating the right side, your fingertips will move up and around toward the right side of your mouth.

- Completely remove your fingertips from the skin after every half-circle is completed, then "step" your fingertips to the next starting place and repeat. Do this until you have covered the entire line of movement.

- You don't need to do the Universal Pass after you finish treating your upper lip. Simply continue to the next part of *Step 3, The Cheeks*.

THE CHEEKS

LOCATION
This large area goes from above the jawline to just below the delicate eye tissue area, and from the side of the nose to the ears.

STARTING POINT
Start where you finished the upper lip section, just above the corner of the mouth.

LINE OF MOVEMENT
While every face is different, you will average two lines of movement here. The first travels along the underside of the cheekbone, toward the ear. The second travels directly over the cheekbone, also toward the ear.

END POINT
The first line will end in front of the center of the ear. The second line will also end in front of the ear, one cup-width above the first end point.

TREATMENT PROCESS
- Attach cup at the starting point and follow the line of movement using lift-and-release and/or moving cups to the end point.
- Repeat this movement three to five times over each cup-width. In all, you will complete six to ten lines of movement.
- Once *Step 3: The Upper Lip and Cheeks* is completed, use lift-and-release and/or moving cups to move the cup down the side of the face toward the jump-off location in front of the ear, then repeat the Universal Pass one to three times before proceeding.
- Continue to *Step 4: The Forehead*.

> **EXCEPTIONS AND WHAT-IFS**
>
> **VERY LOOSE SKIN?** Use the lift-and-release technique. As your skin improves in tone, you can add in moving cups, if desired.
>
> **JAW TENSION?** Do not force the cup to move across an area of resistance. Finish the line of movement with lift-and-release, moving cups, or the Morse Code of Cups technique.
>
> **FACIAL HAIR?** Follow the cup-free recommendations.

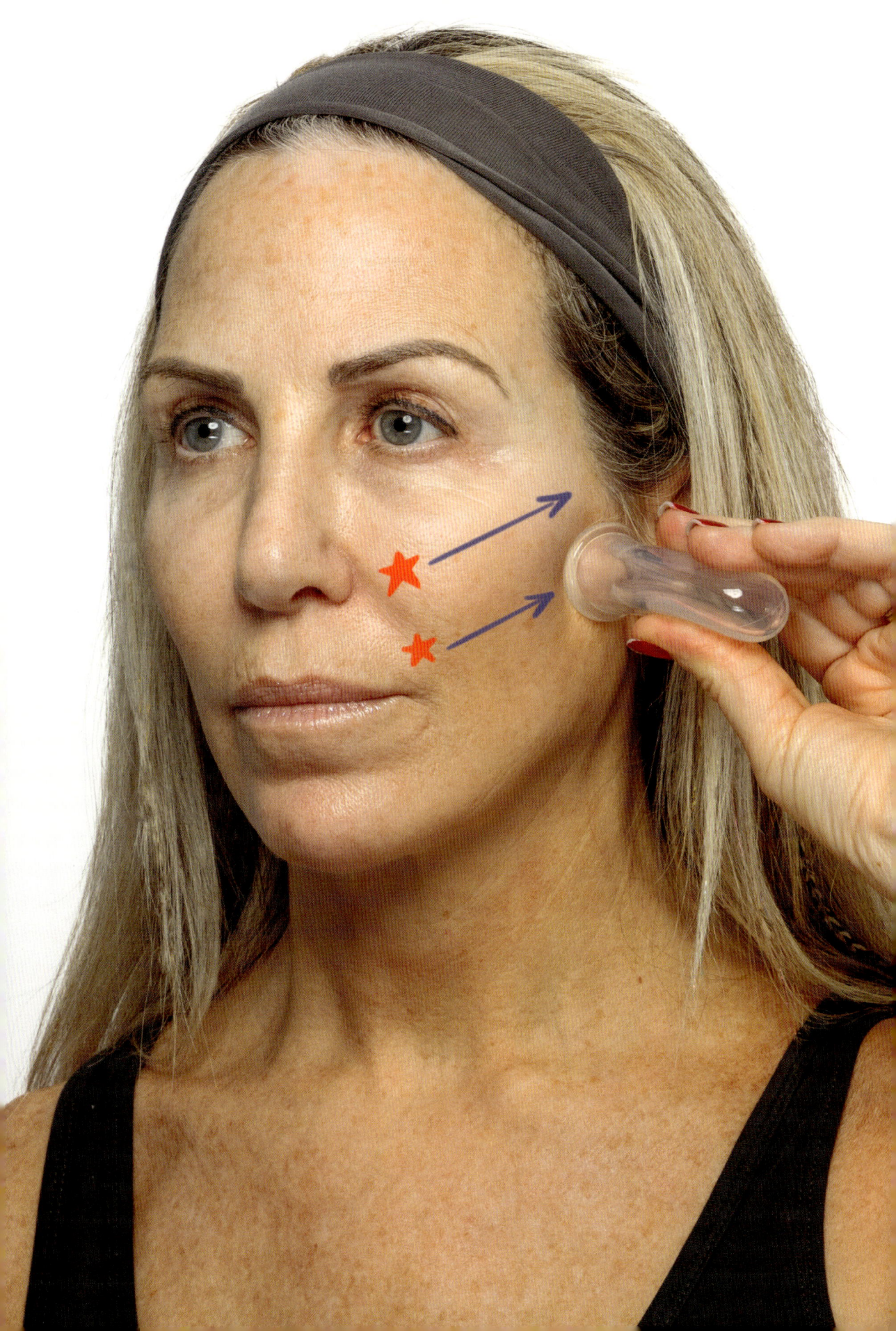

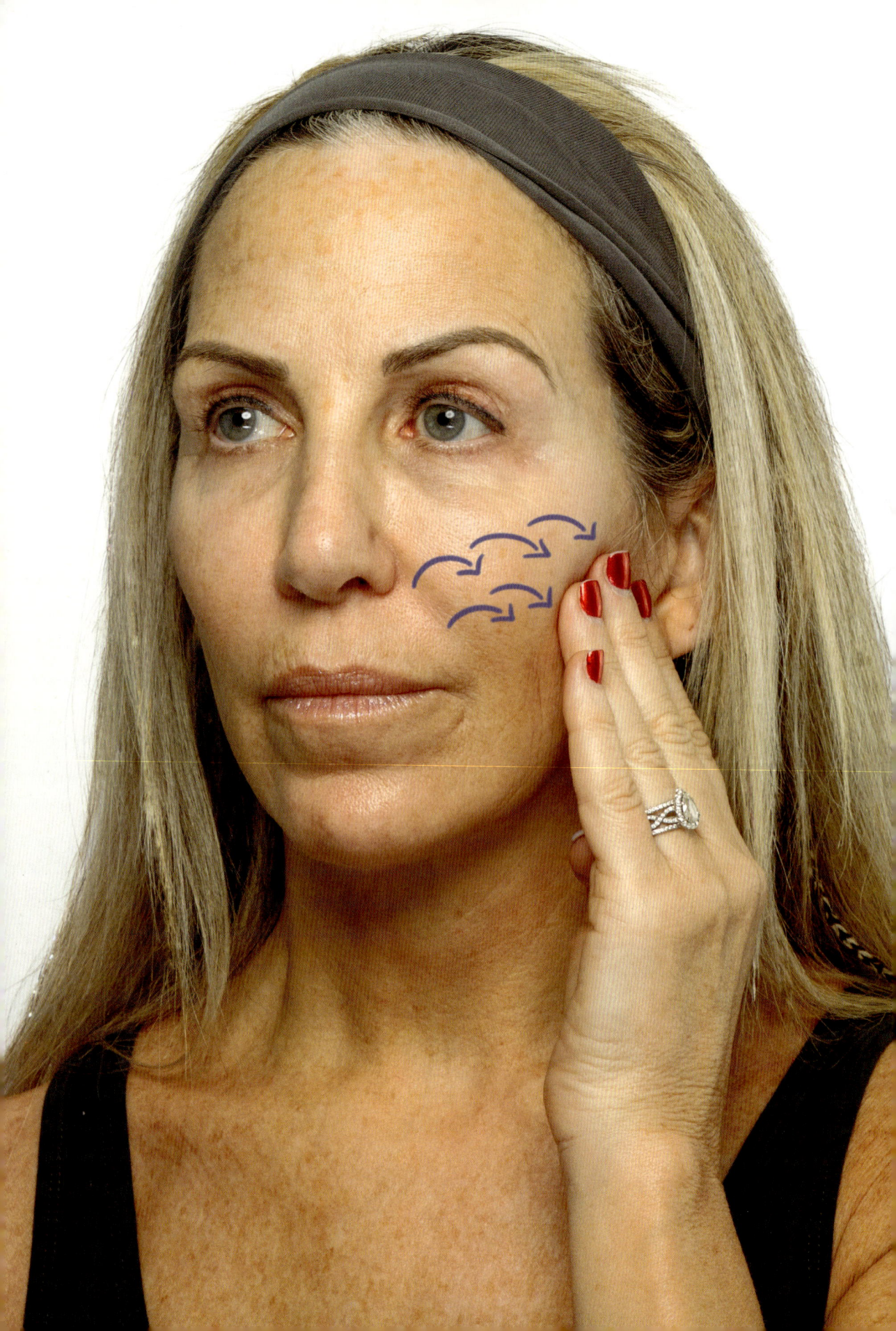

THE CHEEKS

Cup-Free Option

If the cups will not work in this region for whatever reason (facial hair, cosmetic injections, etc.), simply use your fingertips to gently follow the lymph drainage pathways.

TREATMENT PROCESS
Using the same starting point, line of movement and end points as instructed with cups, use your fingertips to create small half-circles across the surface of your skin.

- Begin your fingertip half-circles in the space between the corner of your mouth and the nostril. This is where your upper lip treatment ended, where your smile line wrinkles are.

- As you treat the left side of your face, your fingertips will lightly stretch the skin slightly upward and around toward your left ear. When treating the right side, your fingertips will move up and around toward your right ear.

- Completely remove your fingertips from the skin after every half-circle is completed, then "step" your fingertips to the next starting place and repeat. Do this until you have covered the entire line of movement.

- Repeat the Universal Pass one to three times before proceeding to *Step 4: The Forehead*.

- While every face is different, you will probably do three or four half-circles across each line of movement; if two lines of movement cover your cheek, that equals six or eight half-circles in all. Remember, you are only trying to stimulate the lymph capillaries, so the pressure should be very light.

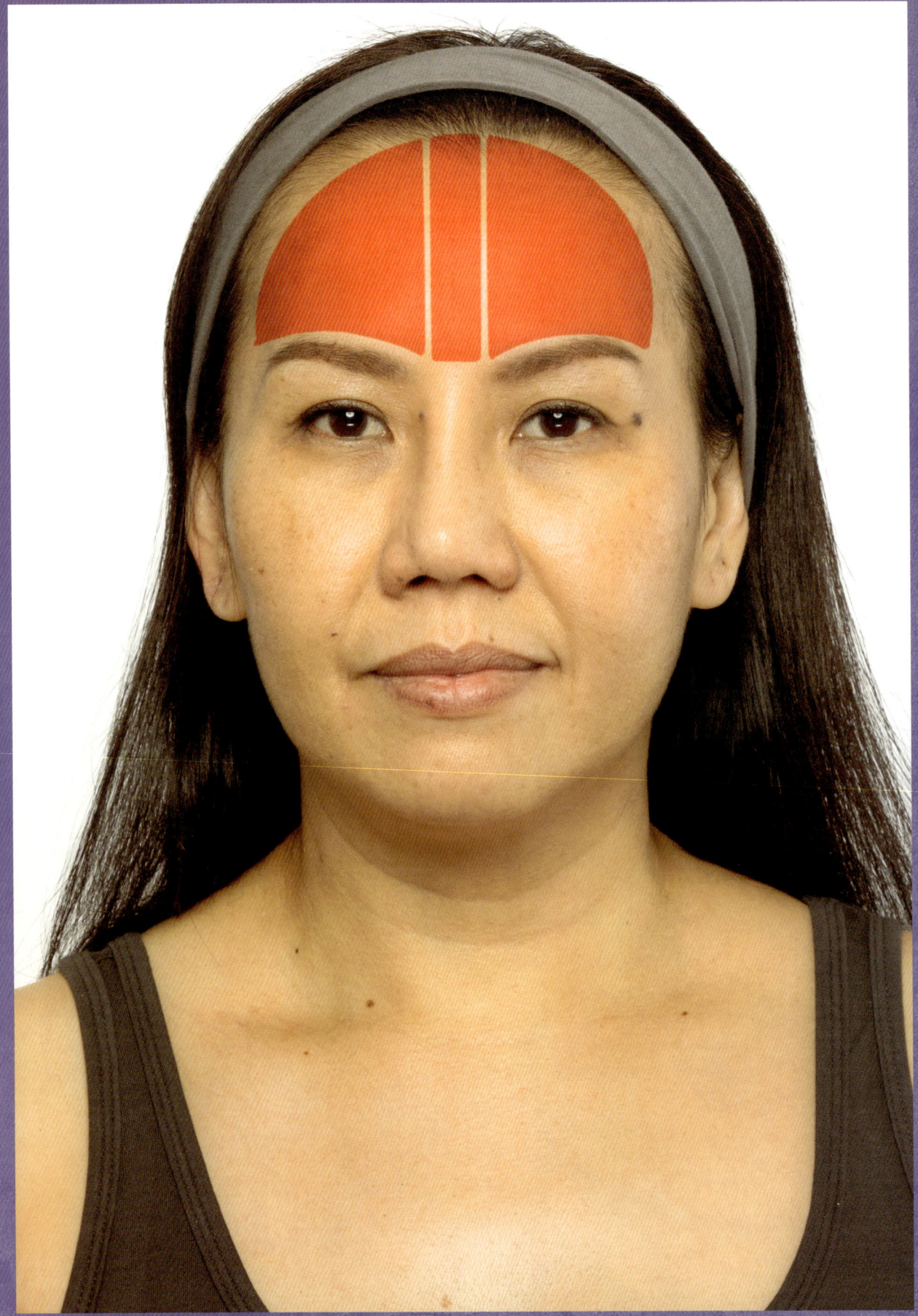

STEP 4
THE FOREHEAD

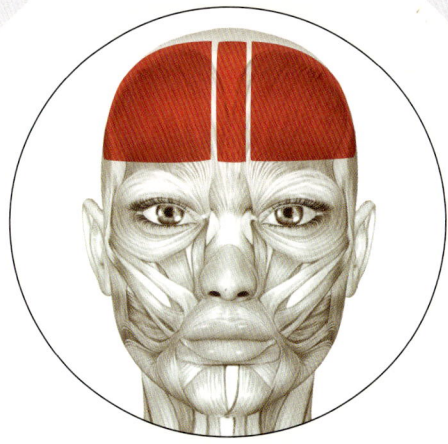

WHY CUP YOUR FOREHEAD?

MANY OF US hold a lot of muscle tension in our forehead, which can contribute to wrinkles, sinus congestion and even headaches.

Cupping is a great way to release tension across the entire forehead. Any wrinkles here will benefit from the softened muscles, and improved circulation brings a healthy glow to the skin. It also offers relief to common sites of sinus congestion and pressure across the forehead.

For the greatest benefits, we divide the cupping treatment for your forehead into two parts: the sinus drainage area and the entire forehead area. Note that there are also cup-free options for both parts.

The small sinus drainage area, which follows the sinus drainage line, both stimulates important lymph drainage vessels and travels over some important therapeutic points for relaxation — enjoy!

> **CUP SIZE**
> Although larger cups work best on your cheek and forehead, tight muscles or boney ridges may not allow you to make an easy connection to the skin in this area. Using a smaller cup may be easier, but use lighter suction and consider lift-and-release only, so you don't get cupping marks!

THE SINUS DRAINAGE AREA

LOCATION
This small region is in the center of the forehead, addressing a straight line from between the eyebrows up toward the hairline. Note that any prominent veins here should be avoided. If necessary, address this area slightly away from this center line (to the left or right, depending on which side of the face you are treating).

STARTING POINT
Start in between your eyebrows, above the top of your nose.

LINE OF MOVEMENT
Follow along the midline of the forehead, upward and toward the hairline.

END POINT
End in the center of the forehead, where your hairline naturally begins.

TREATMENT PROCESS
Be sure to choose a cup size that works for your forehead! (See box on previous page.)

- Attach the cup at the starting point and follow the line of movement using lift-and-release and/or moving cups to the end point.

- Repeat this movement three to five times.

- You don't need to do the Universal Pass after you finish treating the sinus drainage line. Simply continue to the next part of *Step 4, The Entire Forehead.*

> **EXCEPTIONS AND WHAT-IFS**
>
> **SINUS CONGESTION?** Lift-and-release over any sensitive areas. Moving cups will feel great if you're not sensitive! You may add some extra for additional relief; however, don't overwork the area.
>
> **RECENT COSMETIC INJECTIONS?** Don't treat until 30 days post-injection. When you do treat, use lift-and-release or, the closer you are to the procedure, follow the cup-free recommendations.

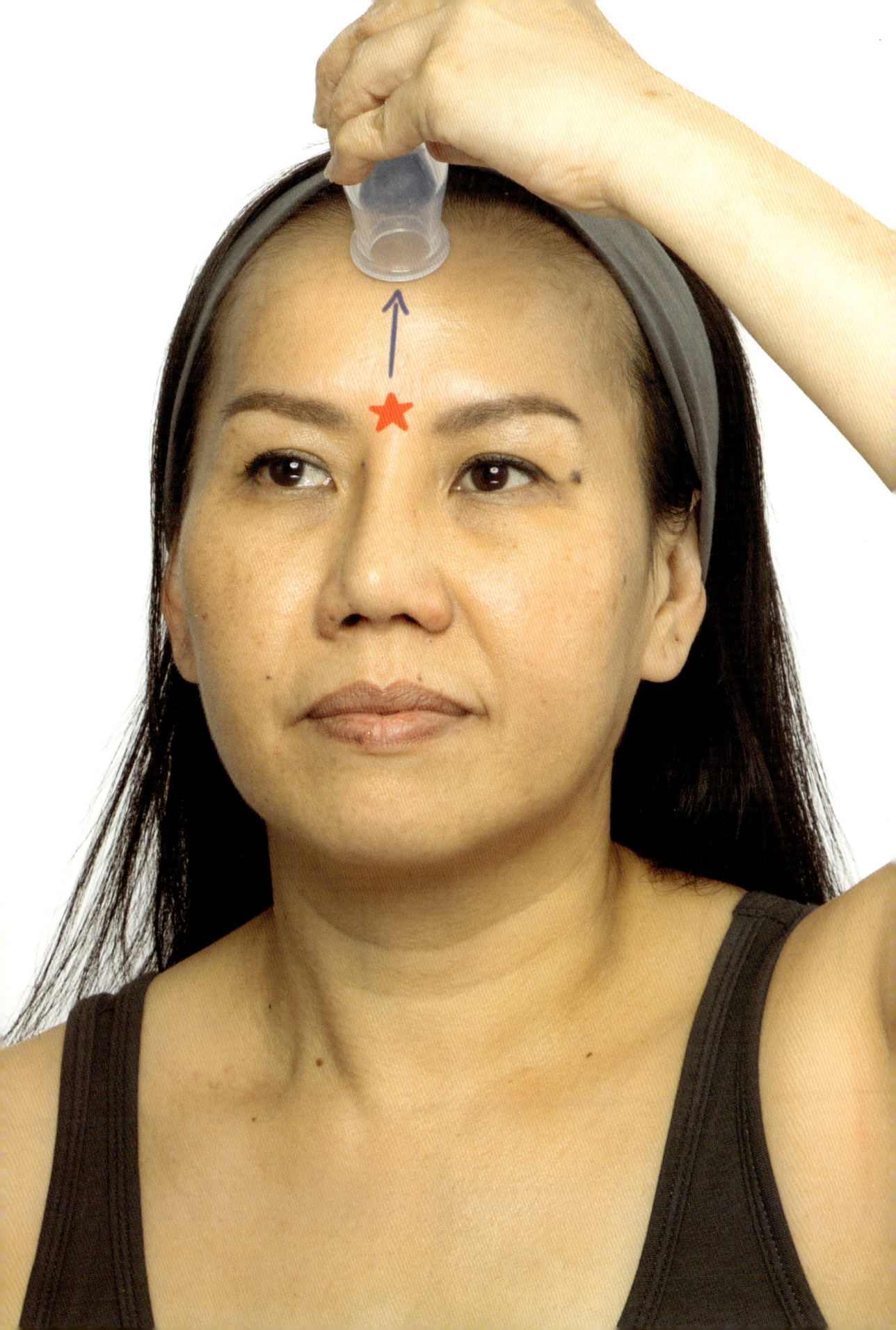

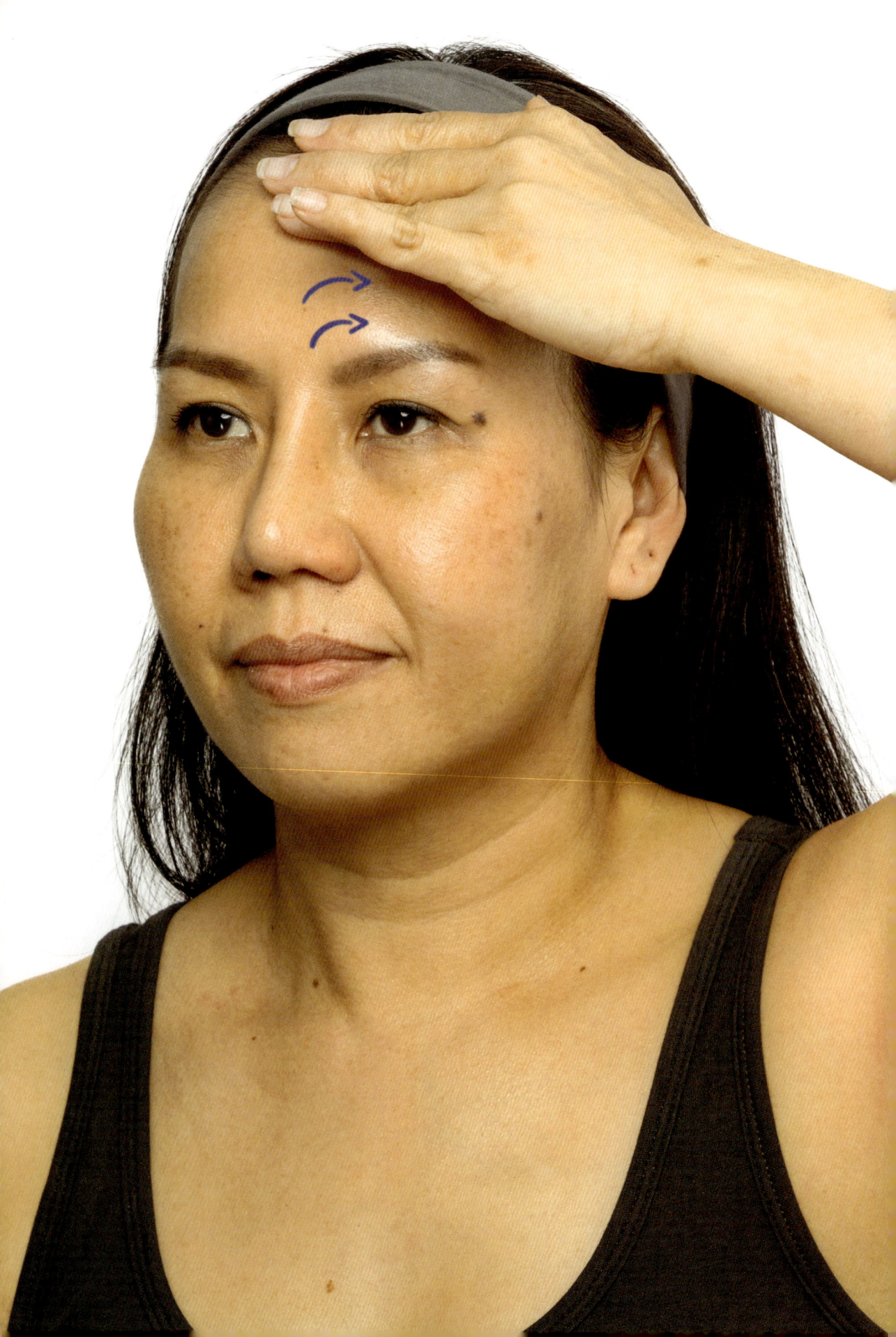

THE SINUS DRAINAGE AREA

Cup-Free Option

If the cups will not work in this region for whatever reason (facial hair, cosmetic injections, etc.), simply use your fingertips to gently follow the lymph drainage pathways.

TREATMENT PROCESS

Using the same starting point, line of movement and end points as instructed with cups, use your fingertips to create small half-circles across the surface of your skin.

▸ Begin your fingertip half-circles in the center of your forehead, in between your eyebrows and above the nose.

▸ As you treat the left side of your face, your fingertips will lightly stretch the skin slightly upward and around toward the left side of your forehead. When treating the right side, your fingertips will move up and around toward the right side of your forehead.

▸ Completely remove your fingertips from the skin after every half-circle is completed, then "step" your fingertips to the next starting place and repeat. Do this until you have covered the entire line of movement.

▸ You don't need to do the Universal Pass after you finish treating the sinus drainage line. Simply continue to the next part of *Step 4, The Entire Forehead*.

THE ENTIRE FOREHEAD

LOCATION
This area covers the rest of the forehead, from the hairline to above the eyebrow. Be sure to avoid any prominent blood vessels, especially in the temple area, as you treat your forehead.

STARTING POINT
Start at the top of the forehead in the centerline, where you finished treating the sinus drainage area.

LINE OF MOVEMENT
This treatment moves from the center of the forehead to the side temple area. With each line of movement, you progress down toward the eyebrow. Your last line of movement will be just above the eyebrow.

END POINT
End above the outer edge of the eyebrow, beside the temple area.

TREATMENT PROCESS

- Attach the cup at the starting point and follow the line of movement using lift-and-release and/or moving cups to the end point.

- Repeat this movement three to five times. The average forehead fits two or three cup-widths; in all, you will complete six to ten lines of movement for the entire forehead area.

- Once *Step 4: The Forehead* is completed, use lift-and-release and/or moving cups to move the cup down the side of the face toward the jump-off location in front of the ear, then repeat the Universal Pass one to three times before proceeding.

- Continue to *Step 5: The Eyes*.

EXCEPTIONS AND WHAT-IFS

SINUS CONGESTION? Lift-and-release over any sensitive areas. Moving cups will feel great if you're not sensitive!

RECENT COSMETIC INJECTIONS? Don't treat until 30 days post-injection. When you do treat, use lift-and-release or, the closer you are to the procedure, follow the cup-free recommendations.

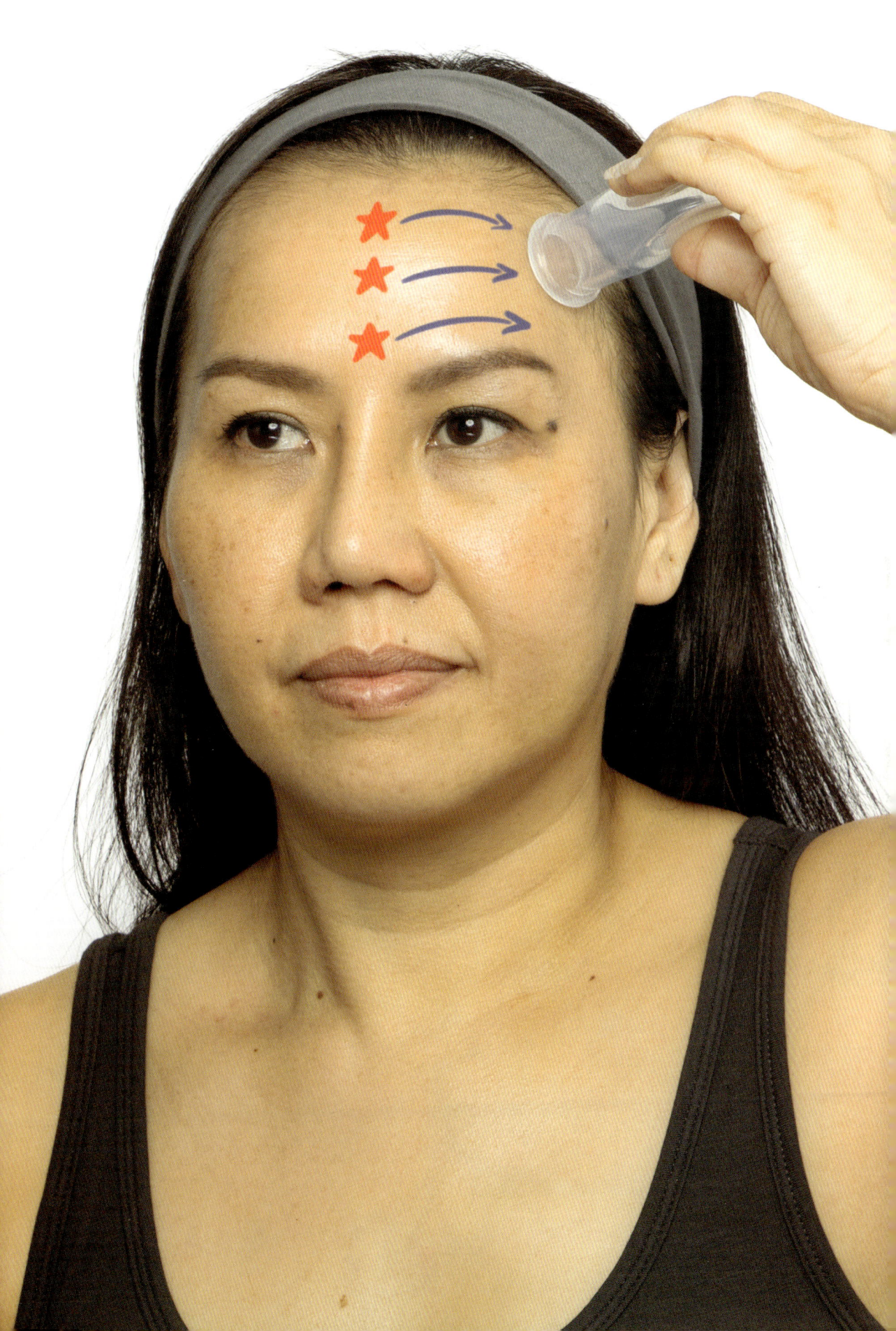

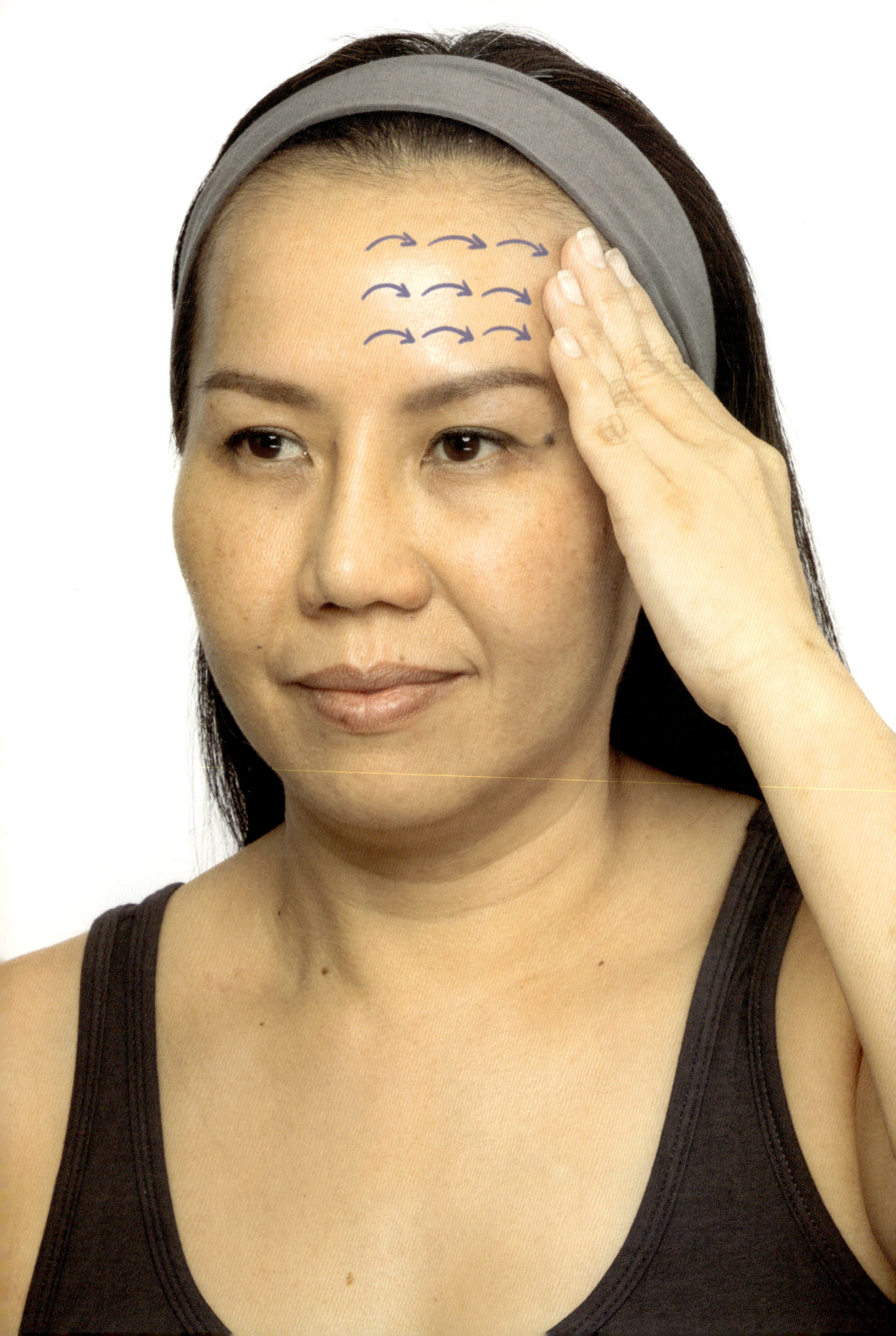

THE ENTIRE FOREHEAD

Cup-Free Option

If the cups will not work in this region for whatever reason (facial hair, cosmetic injections, etc.), simply use your fingertips to gently follow the lymph drainage pathways.

TREATMENT PROCESS
Using the same starting point, line of movement and end point as instructed with cups, use your fingertips to create small half-circles across the surface of your skin.

- Begin your fingertip half-circles in the center of the forehead at the natural hairline; this is where the sinus drainage area treatment just ended.

- As you treat the left side of your face, your fingertips will lightly stretch the skin slightly upward and around toward the left temple area. When treating the right side, your fingertips will move up and around toward the right temple area.

- Completely remove your fingertips from the skin after every half-circle is completed, then "step" your fingertips to the next starting place and repeat. Do this until you have covered the entire line of movement.

- Repeat the Universal Pass one to three times before proceeding to *Step 5: The Eyes*.

- While every face is different, you will probably do three or four half-circles across each line of movement; if two lines of movement cover your forehead region, that is six or eight half-circles total. Remember, you are only trying to stimulate the lymph capillaries, so the pressure should be very light.

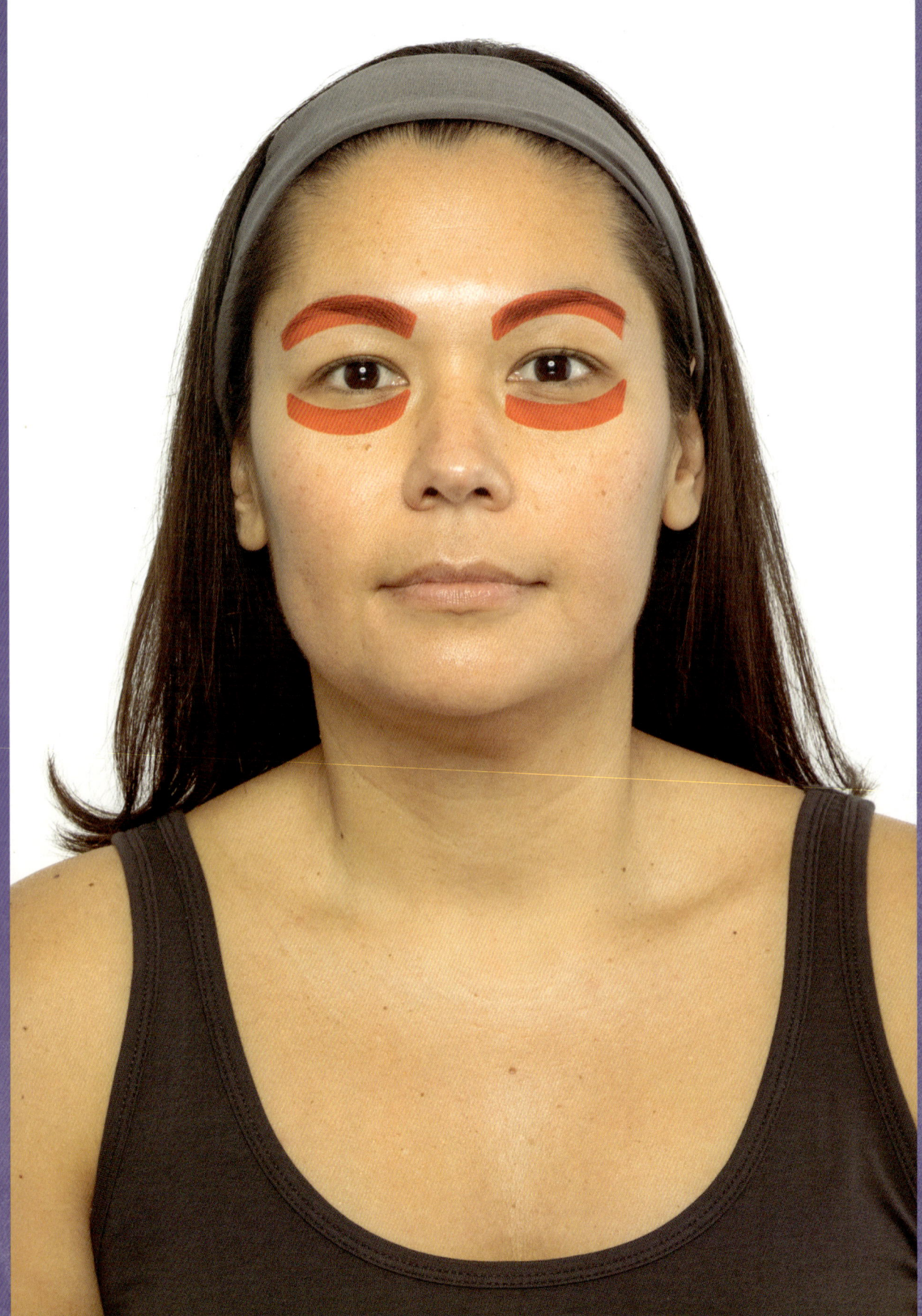

STEP 5
THE EYE AREA

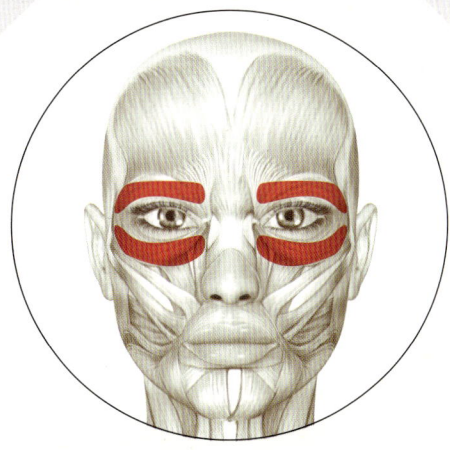

WHY CUP YOUR EYES?

THE THINNEST, MOST DELICATE SKIN of the entire body is around the eyes. Often the first location to experience cosmetic changes, this is a common site of loose skin and wrinkle lines.

Cupping around the eyes is very delicate, too, and must be done with the utmost attention to detail. A little goes a long way here, so be sure to use very light suction with only the lift-and-release technique here — no moving cups! When done correctly, the toning effects are incredible.

For the greatest benefits, we divide the cupping treatment for your eyes into two parts: under the eye and above the eye.

Note that there are also cup-free options for both parts. With or without cups, treatment in the eye area can be extremely beneficial for everyone.

> **DELICATE EYE TISSUE**
> **CAUTION:** Until you become comfortable with the cupping process, make this a cup-free location. The benefits will still be great.

UNDER THE EYE

Remember, do not slide the cup in this delicate eye tissue area.

LOCATION
This is a very small, delicate region. Be sure to avoid making contact with the lower eyelid near the eyelashes; stay closer to the region at the top of the cheek.

STARTING POINT
Start at the side of the nose, at the bottom of the delicate eye tissue area.

LINE OF MOVEMENT
This treatment moves from the starting point at the side of the nose, along the underside of the eye, toward the outer edge of the eye.

END POINT
End at the outer edge of the eye, still underneath the eye, at the bottom of the delicate eye tissue area.

TREATMENT PROCESS
Be sure to use a small cup when you treat your eye area.

- Using only lift-and-release, attach the cup at the starting point and follow along the line of movement to the end point.

- Repeat this line of movement three to five times.

- You don't need to do the Universal Pass after you finish treating under the eye. Simply continue to the next part of *Step 5, Above the Eye.*

> **EXCEPTIONS AND WHAT-IFS**
>
> **RECENT COSMETIC INJECTIONS?** Don't treat until 30 days post-injection. When you do treat, use lift-and-release or, the closer you are to the procedure, follow the cup-free recommendations.
>
> **VERY LOOSE SKIN?** Follow the recommended cup-free option.

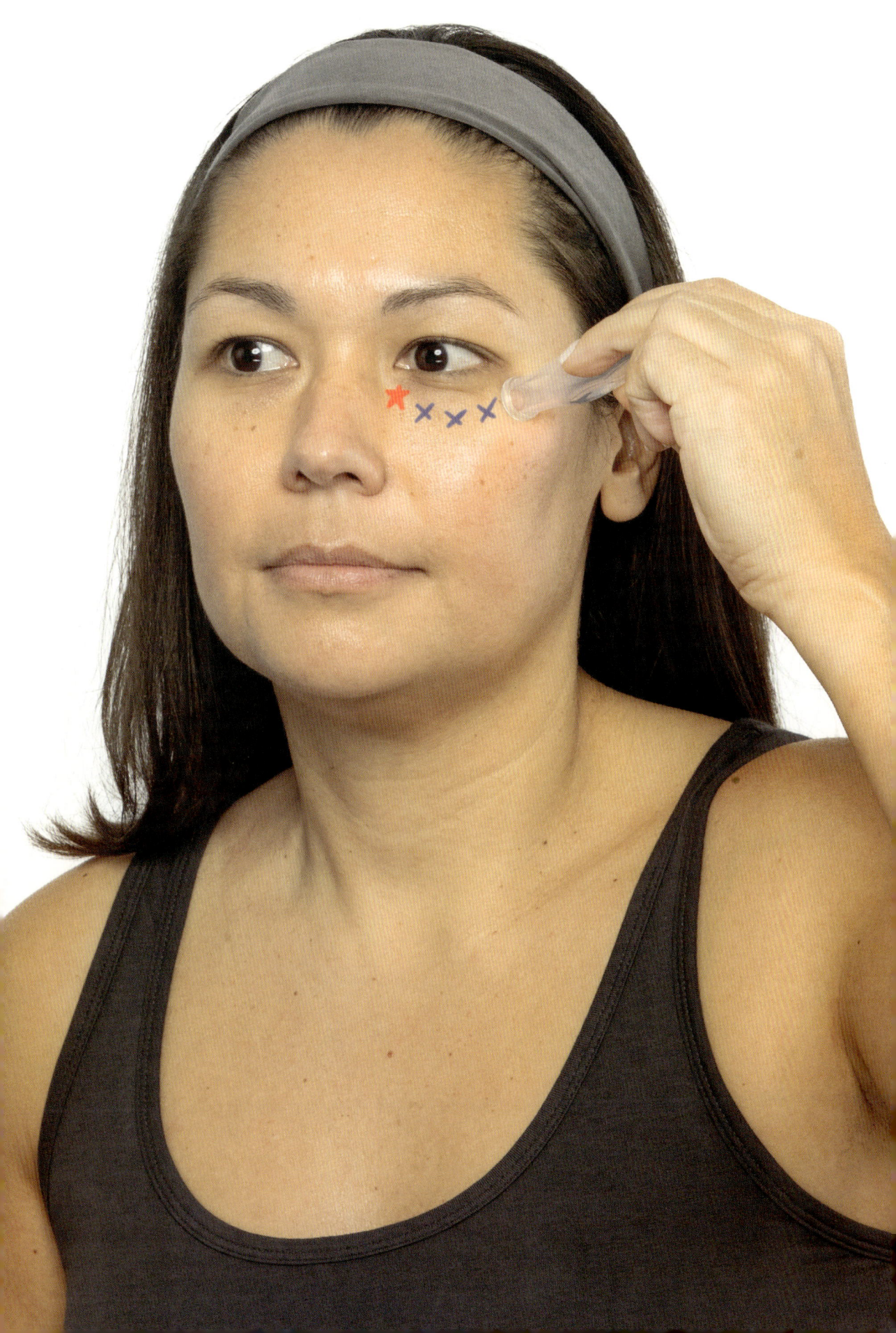

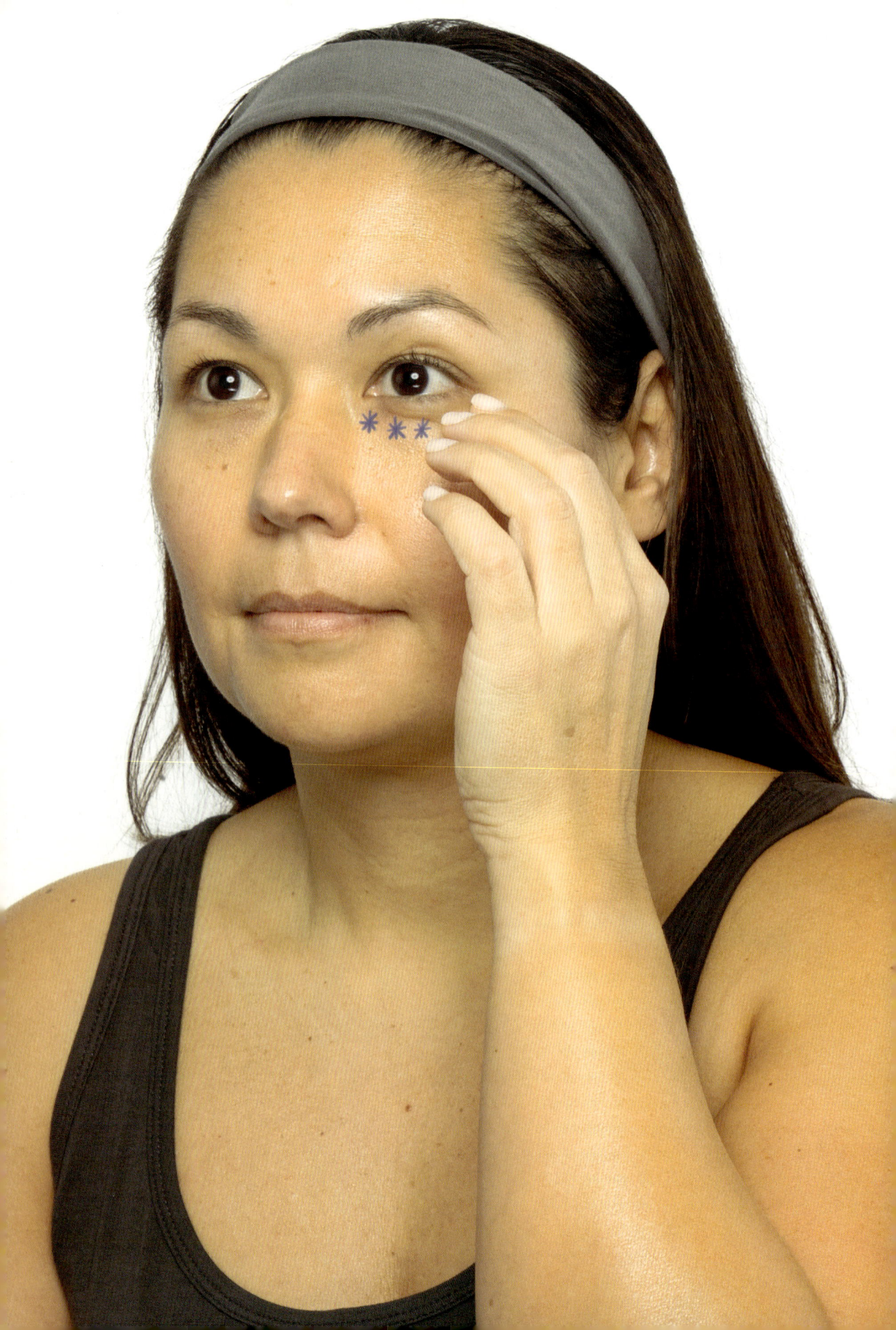

UNDER THE EYE

Cup-Free Option

If the cups will not work in this region for whatever reason (facial hair, cosmetic injections, etc.), simply use your fingertips to gently follow the lymph drainage pathways.

> Because of the delicacy of the eye area, this cup-free option is highly recommended and very popular.

TREATMENT PROCESS

Using the same starting point, line of movement and end point as instructed with cups, use your fingertips to gently tap along the underside of the eyes. This technique is extra beneficial for toning the delicate skin here.

- Using three or four fingertips, one after the other and progressing out to the sides, begin to gently tap the skin's surface quickly and repeatedly throughout the area. We call this method of application the "piano move."

- As you treat the left side of your face, use your fingertips to repetitively tap from the center outward, ending at the outer edge of your eye. When treating the right side, repetitively tap from the center and out toward the outer edge of your eye.

- You don't need to do the Universal Pass after you finish treating under the eye. Simply continue to the next part of *Step 5, Above the Eye*.

ABOVE THE EYE

LOCATION
This step safely addresses the area above the eye by treating the eyebrow. While cupping the eyebrow can be challenging, working along this line will benefit the delicate skin above the eye and eyelid, the ridge of the eyebrow, the sinus areas and the lower areas of the forehead. If a thicker eyebrow or a bony ridge below the brow will not allow you to attach the cup easily, do not get frustrated — simply follow the cup-free recommendations instead.

STARTING POINT
Start at the inner edge of the eyebrow, directly above the delicate eye tissue area.

LINE OF MOVEMENT
This treatment moves across the entire eyebrow region, from the center out toward the temple area.

END POINT
Stop at the outer edge of the eyebrow, just before the temple area.

TREATMENT PROCESS
Be sure you are using a cup that fits your eyebrow; if no cup works, follow the cup-free recommendations.

▸ Attach cup at the starting point and follow the line of movement using lift-and-release and/or moving cups to the end point. Unless there is little to no eyebrow hair, most eyebrows will be lift-and-release only.

▸ Repeat this movement three to five times.

▸ Once *Step 5: The Eye Area* is completed, use lift-and-release and/or moving cups to move the cup down the side of the face toward the jump-off location in front of the ear, then repeat the Universal Pass one to three times. You have finished the entire treatment!

> **EXCEPTIONS AND WHAT-IFS**
> **SINUS CONGESTION?** Lift-and-release over any sensitive areas.

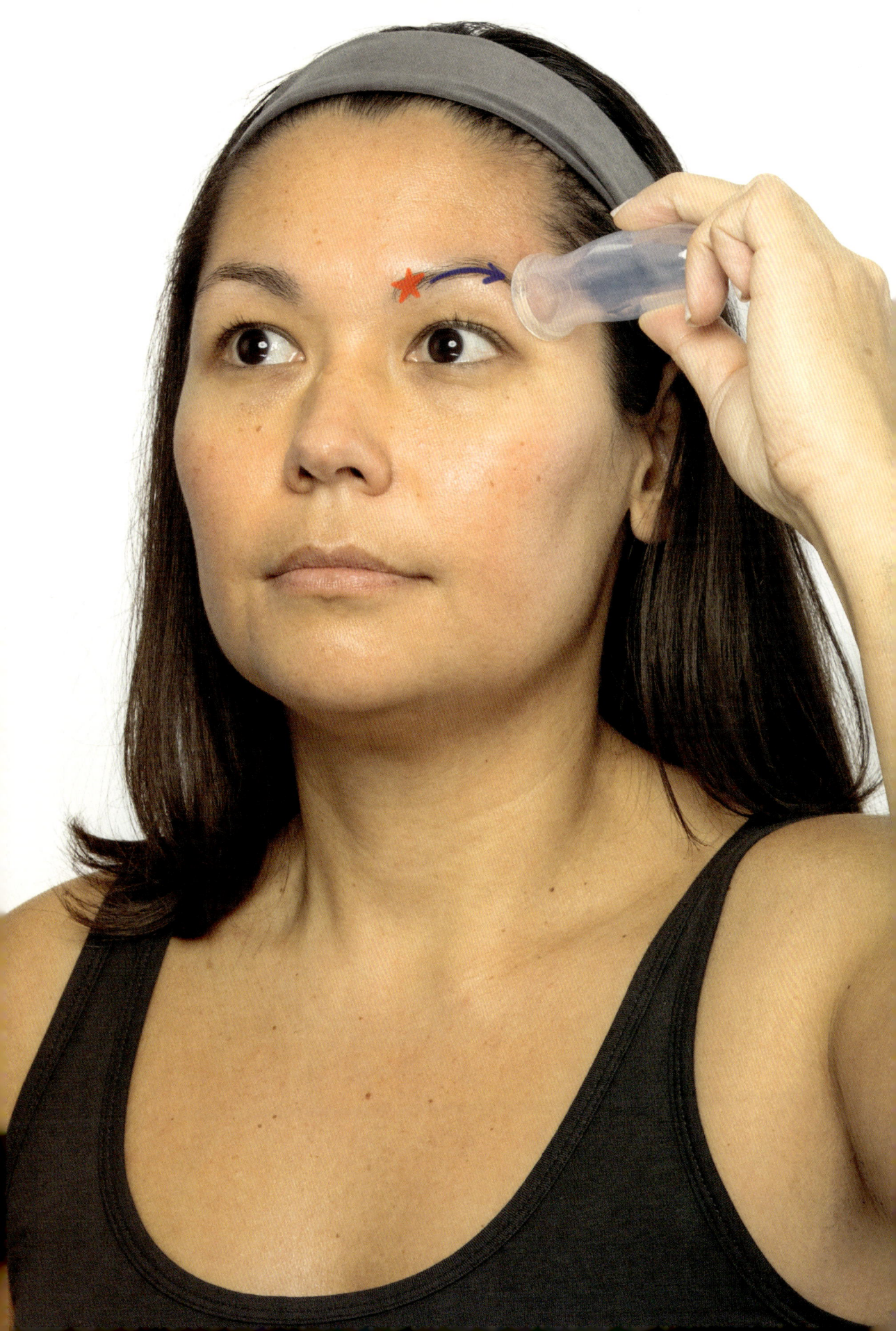

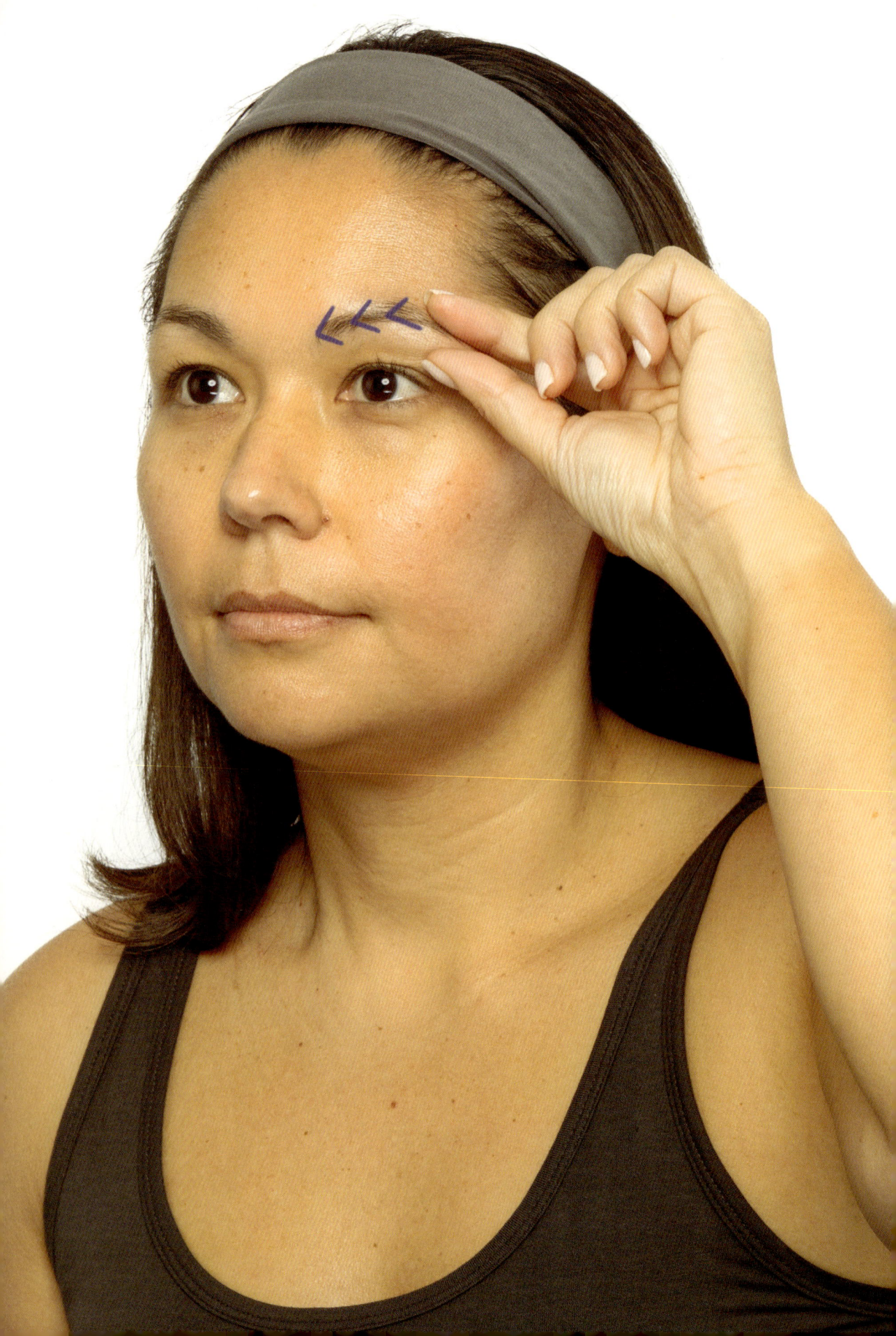

ABOVE THE EYE

Cup-Free Option

If the cups will not work in this region for whatever reason (facial hair, cosmetic injections, etc.), simply use your fingertips to gently follow the lymph drainage pathways. This cup-free option also offers sinus congestion relief.

> Because of the delicacy of the eye area, this cup-free option is highly recommended and very popular.

TREATMENT PROCESS

Using the same starting point, line of movement and end point as instructed with cups, use your fingertips to pinch the eyebrows from the center and progress outward.

- Using your thumb and index finger, gently pinch your eyebrows one pinch at a time, progressing out to the side.

- As you treat the left side of your face, your pinches will progress from the center outward, ending at the outer edge of your left eyebrow. When treating the right side, your pinches will progress from the center outward, ending at the outer edge of your right eyebrow.

- Once *Step 5: The Eye Area* is completed, slide your flattened fingertips down the side of your face, then repeat the Universal Pass one to three times. You have finished the entire treatment!

THE FACE-CUPPING MAP

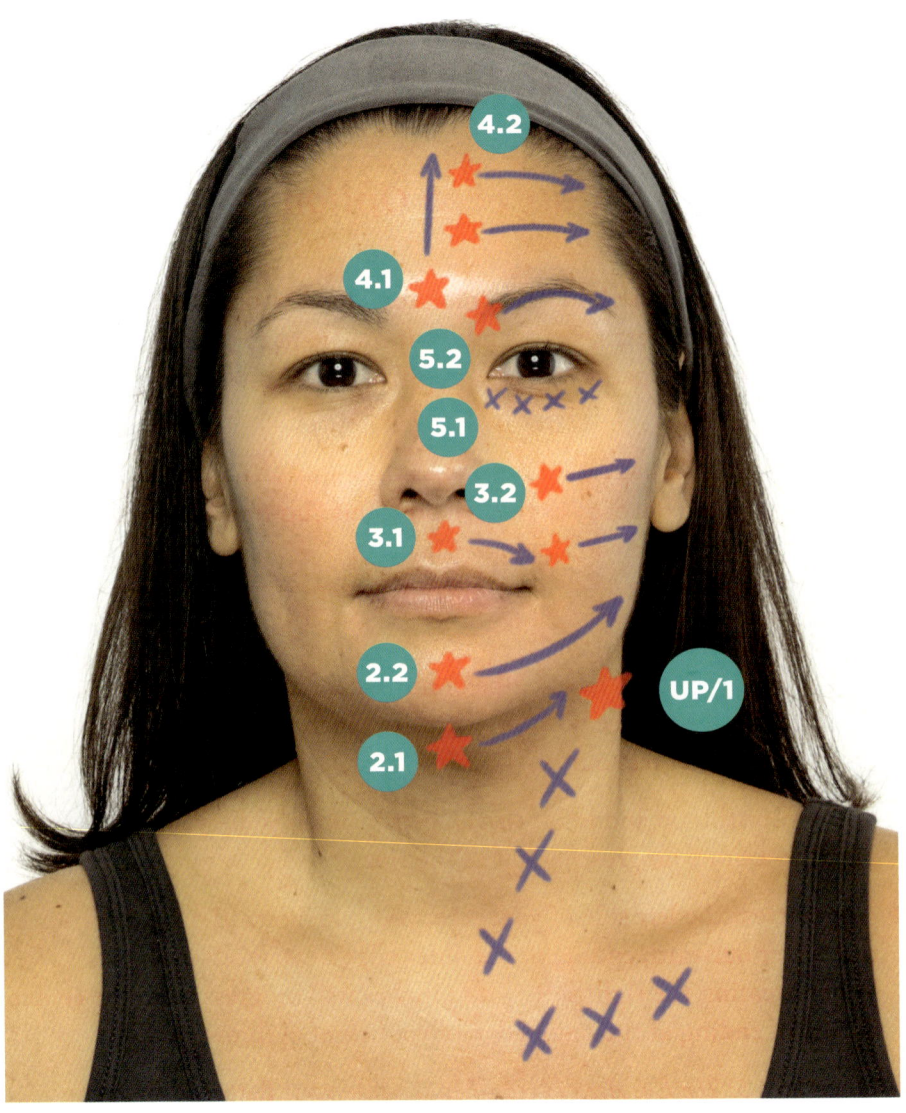

LEGEND

UP/1	Universal Pass / Step 1: The Neck and Upper Chest (pages 98/106)
2.1	Step 2: Below the Jawline (page 112)
2.2	Step 2: Above the Jawline (page 116)
3.1	Step 3: The Upper Lip (page 122)
3.2	Step 3: The Cheeks (page 126)
4.1	Step 4: The Sinus Drainage Area (page 132)
4.2	Step 4: The Entire Forehead (page 136)
5.1	Step 5: Under the Eye (page 142)
5.2	Step 5: Above the Eye (page 146)

REMEMBER THESE TREATMENT POINTERS

- Use moving cups or lift-and-release techniques — no stationary cups.

- Pressure should be light.

- Cup should be proportional to the face and larger in size.

- The application should be slow, rhythmic and repetitive.

- Treat the entire face evenly, one cup-width at a time.

- Start on the left side.

- Follow the step-by-step instructions as written.

- Repeat the Universal Pass at the end of each step as directed in the instructions.

- Look for the exceptions.

- Use only the lift-and-release technique in the front of the neck — no moving cups.

CHAPTER 8

AFTER YOUR FACIAL CUPPING TREATMENT

Products to Apply
154

Make a Treatment Plan
158

CONGRATULATIONS on learning how to do facial cupping for yourself! In this section, I'd like to offer a few after-care suggestions to complement your treatment. We will discuss products to apply and creating a treatment plan to achieve your best self-care results.

Products to Apply

FIRST, BEFORE YOU apply any products on your skin, I recommend that you clean your face immediately after your treatment. Although many oils are great for your skin, cleaning your face after you have finished your facial cupping treatment will remove the oil and any pore gunk that may have been loosened and "vacuumed" from your pores. It also prepares your skin for whatever great products you want to apply afterward.

APPLY YOUR FAVORITE SKINCARE PRODUCTS. Since cupping boosts circulation and gently dilates your pores, as your circulation recedes any product you apply afterward will be absorbed more efficiently. Whether you apply your favorite serum, quality face oil or a good moisturizer, any product you choose will have a more penetrating effect when applied immediately following your facial cupping treatment.

OPTION: APPLY A FACE MASK! With the boosted skin activity that follows cupping, what better time to use a cleansing, tightening or toning face mask? And apply your favorite skincare products after you remove the mask.

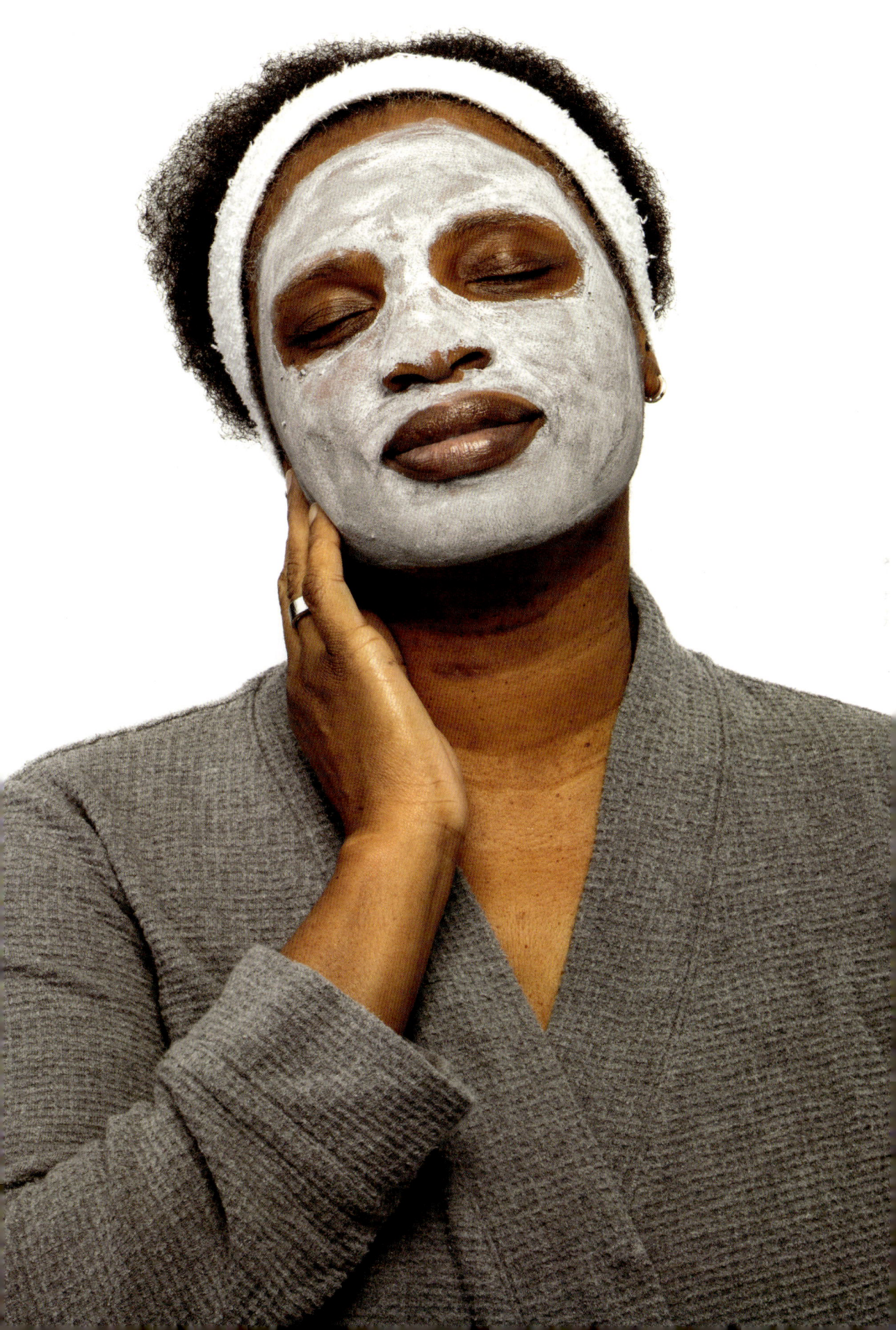

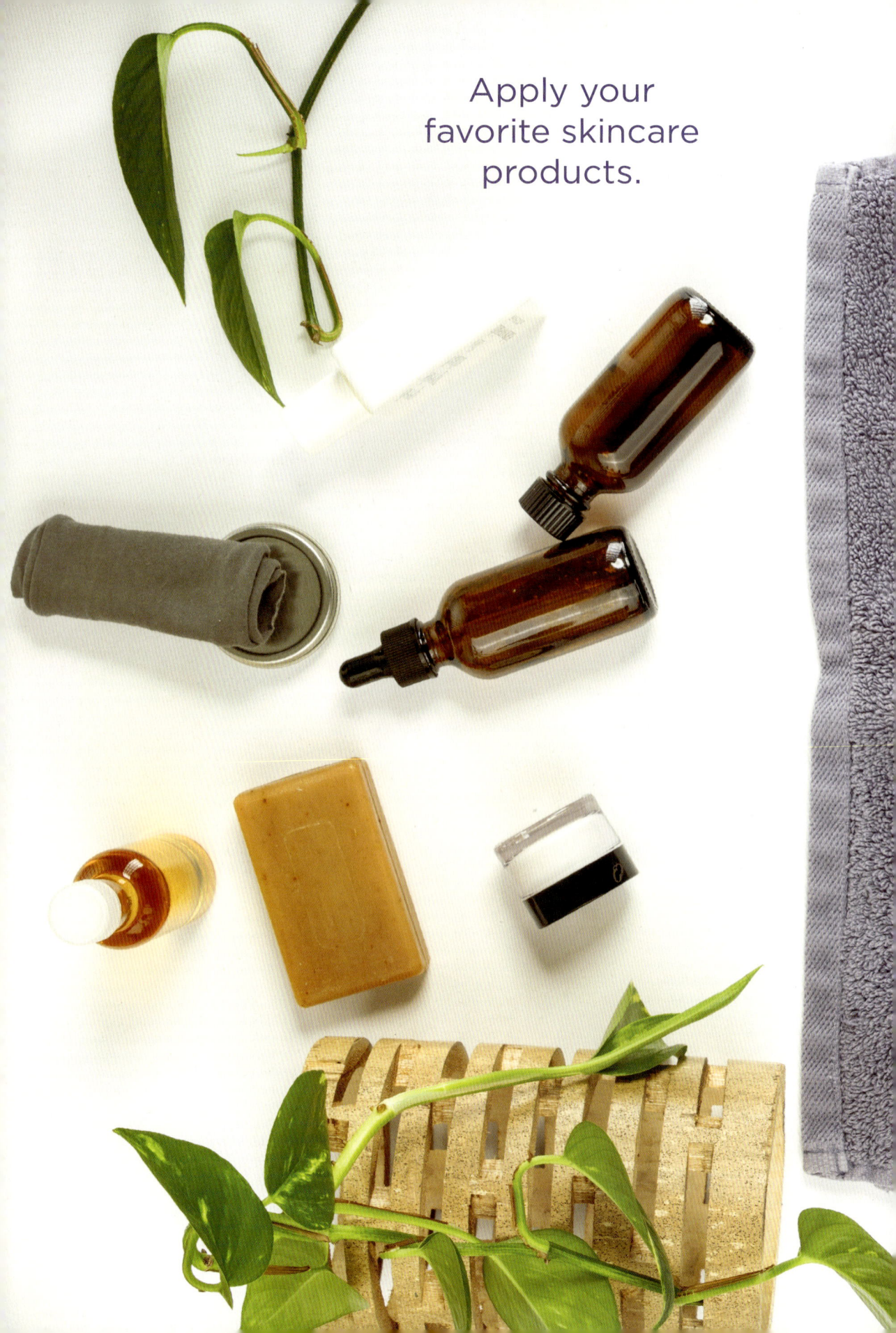
Apply your favorite skincare products.

WHAT TO AVOID:

- **AVOID EXCESSIVE HEAT OR COLD APPLICATIONS IMMEDIATELY FOLLOWING YOUR TREATMENT.** While a warm compress may feel good and help to remove the oil, make sure it isn't too hot. Extreme heat after such a circulation-boosting treatment can be too stimulating for the skin, possibly creating swelling or skin irritation. Conversely, if you are a fan of cool compresses or other cool temperature applications after such a treatment, just be sure it isn't too cold, as that could shock your face skin and pores.

- **AVOID STRONG EXFOLIATION OR OTHER AGGRESSIVE SKIN TREATMENTS.** Even though facial cupping is gentle, it is a very powerful treatment for your skin. Let your skin rest after your treatment. Exfoliation can be irritating, and other treatments such as scraping or guasha can also overstimulate the delicate face skin. When facial cupping treatment is included as part of a professional facial, it is generally followed only by the application of a face mask or final skincare products.

Make a Treatment Plan

HOW OFTEN can you give yourself a facial cupping treatment? I recommend that you treat yourself no more than every 48 hours. While the results are amazing, if you were to do this every day, some adverse reactions could occur.

First, since cups affect fluid levels in the tissues, cupping too much could create swelling. And if the tissue swells too much, over time this can cause circulation issues. Furthermore, if swelling occurs and then dissipates repeatedly, this could distort the skin, causing it to sag.

Also, if you cup the face daily, you will most likely cause cupping marks, as the delicate facial tissues need those 48 hours to fully process not only the fluid movements within the circulatory system, but also what has been stirred up within the muscle tissue, too. Wrinkles are a clear indication of adhesions; if you cup over them too much — day after day — cupping marks will most likely surface.

RECOMMENDATION: Pick one or two days (maximum) per week to schedule a treatment. Consider this to be a self-care date with yourself. I personally like "Wellness Wednesdays" and do my best to treat my face every Wednesday.

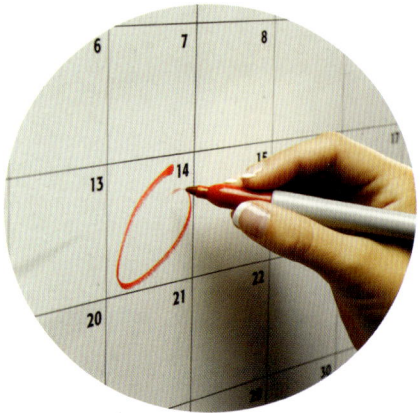

PLANNING OPTION: Schedule one month for a treatment series. Plan to do this treatment once or twice each week for one month; be sure to take photos before you start and after you have finished. You will see (and feel) some wonderful changes, and that will motivate you to keep doing the cupping!

In my clinical practice, some people come in for the treatment series before major events like weddings or reunions, while others simply come in for their monthly bodywork treatment and add this facial cupping into every monthly visit. You will be the best judge of what works best for you and your needs. Have fun with it — don't overdo it — and you will be forever a fan of facial cupping, too!

> ### HOW LONG DO THE RESULTS LAST?
> Every person will have different results, and cupping results are most responsive when you follow all recommendations for application, timing and frequency. Cupping results are cumulative and lasting. Yes, the clock of time keeps ticking forward, but with regular treatments, facial cupping is one of the most effective, natural treatments to ensure a long, beautiful life for your face. I hope that you are excited to get to work on yourself!

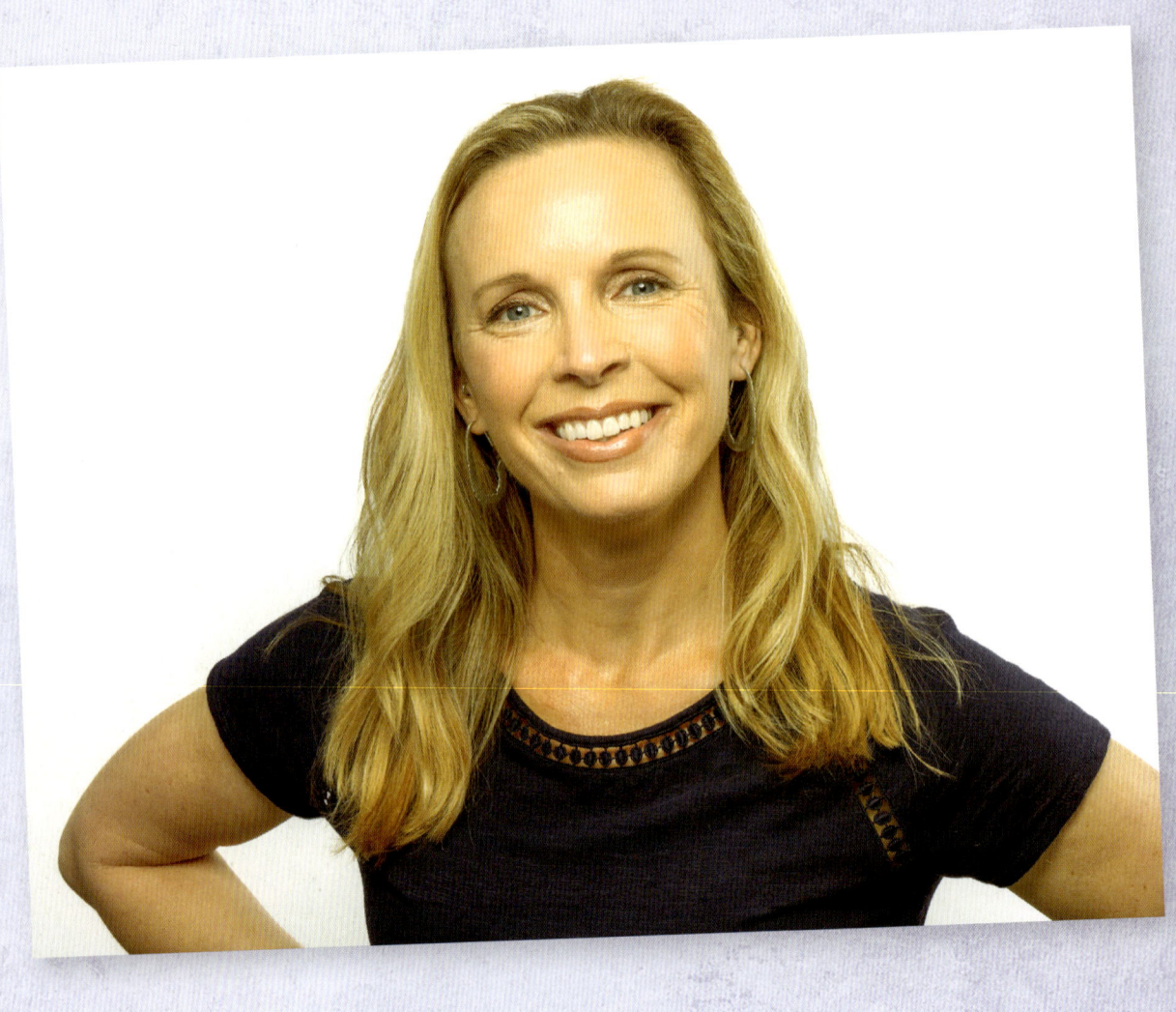

The Full Potential of Therapeutic Cupping for Skin Health

MY STORY

MY PERSONAL STORY of facial cupping is what brought me to be the professional bodyworker and cupping instructor I am today.

At age 18, I suffered a major car accident that left me with many injuries, including a very large scar across the left side of my face. My face received dozens of stitches to repair it, and within the layers of healing skin remained bits of glass and sand from the impact. While I was thankful to be alive, as a teenage girl, knowing my face was disfigured was shocking, to say the least. The jaw pain and dysfunction that accompanied such an injury was just as traumatic.

I first experienced cups on my face almost three years later. While it was an emotional experience for me to let someone touch my face with cups, the sensations and the visible results were quite dramatic in a positive, comforting way. I began practicing facial cupping on a regular basis, following the natural lymph drainage pathways and learning what worked best for such a treatment. Over many sessions, my scar became less visible and the pain in my face diminished. Over time, some of the glass and sand that was stuck in my face came to the surface and was successfully removed.

My personal experience motivated me to become the cupping instructor I am. I have a strong desire to share this powerful information with as many people as I can. Every time I share my history, people have a hard time even identifying where my scar is until I point it out; cupping has helped heal my skin that much!

This treatment offers remarkable benefits to the skin on so many levels, and it is truly one of the most amazing treatments I have ever received. Because of this, I offer it in clinical settings for not only cosmetic enhancement, but for all the other health and functional benefits cupping the face offers.

From one of the most traumatic incidents of my life came a gift I want to share with the world. I hope you enjoy your facial cupping treatment and all the magic that it truly offers.

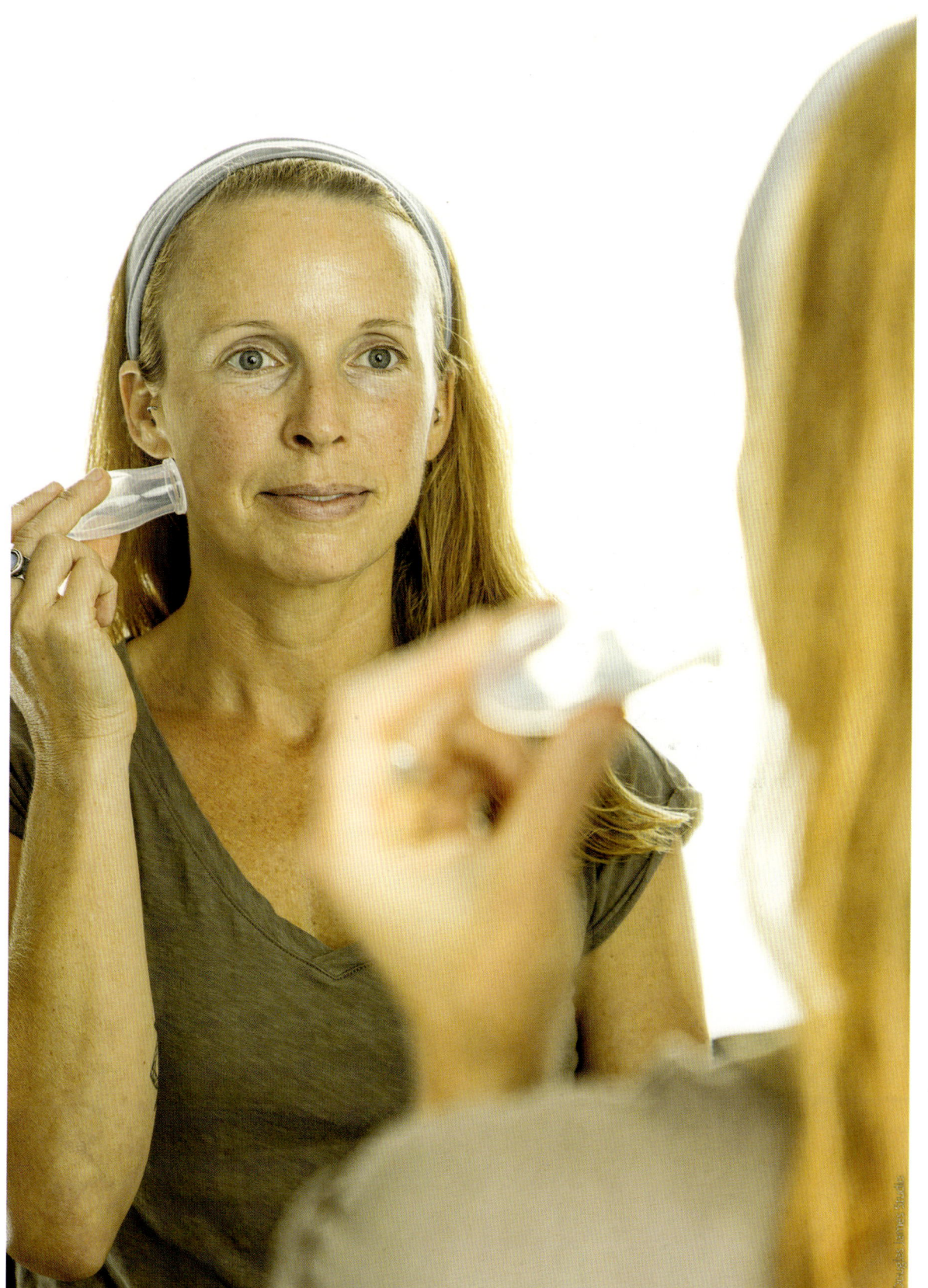

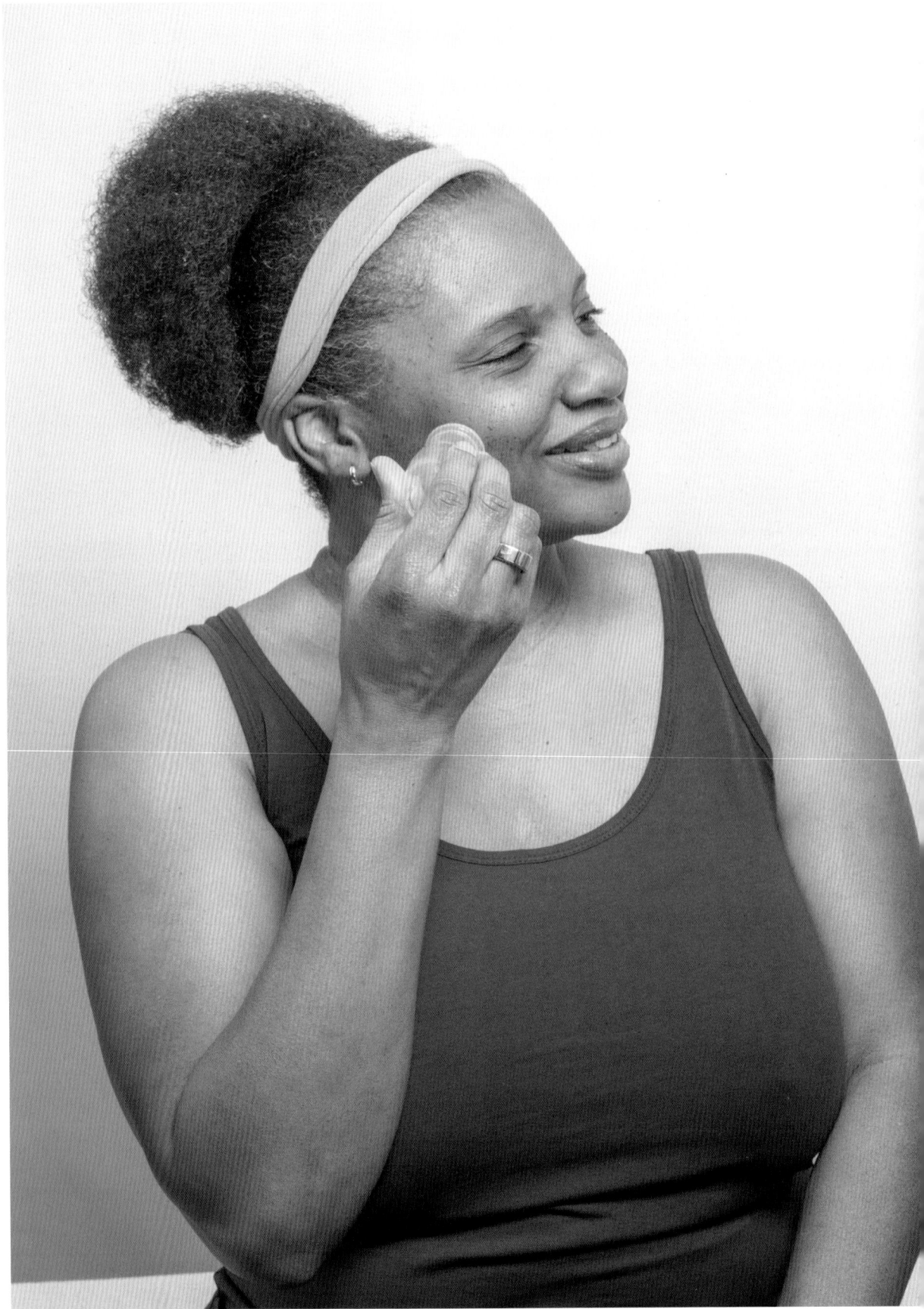

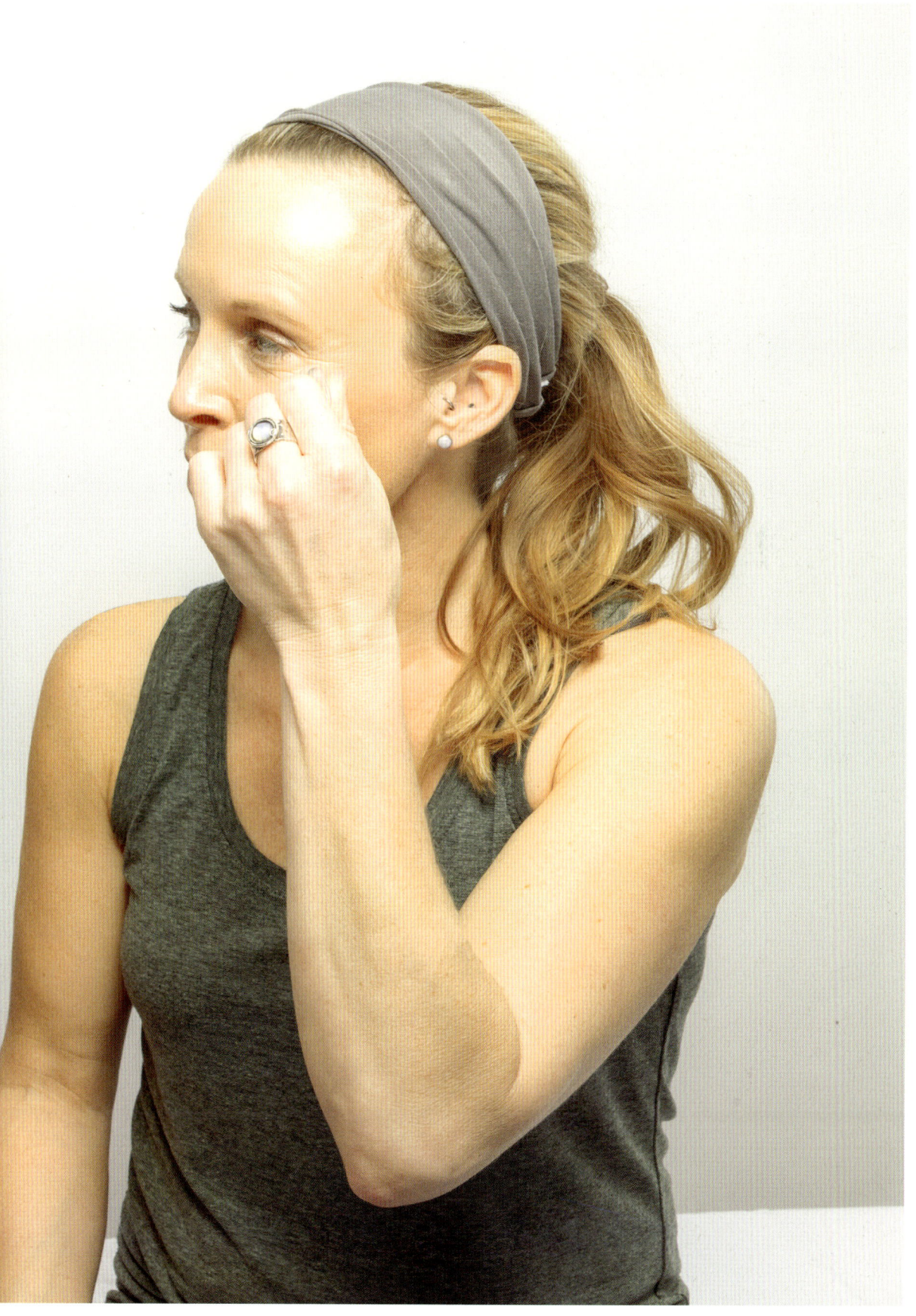

I hope you enjoy your facial cupping treatment and all the magic that it truly offers.

REFERENCES AND RESOURCES

BOOKS

Amato, L., H. Bickmore, J. Doyle, M. Nielsen, L. Sarfati, J. Schlaiss, and L. Todd. 2020. *Milady Standard Esthetics*. 12th ed. Cengage Publishing

Földi, M., and R. Strössenreuther. 2005. *Foundations of Manual Lymph Drainage*. 3rd ed. Elsevier Mosby Publishing

Gilmartin, Shannon. 2017. *The Guide to Modern Cupping Therapy: Your Step-by-Step Source for Vacuum Therapy*. Robert Rose Publishing

Wittlinger, H., D. Wittlinger, A. Wittlinger, and M. Wittlinger. Translated by R. Gutberlet. 2019. *Dr. Vodder's Manual Lymph Drainage: A Practical Guide*. 2nd ed. Thieme Publishings Stuttgart

ARTICLES

Al-Bedah, A.M.N., I.S. Elsubai, N.A. Qureshi, T.S. Aboushanab, G.I.M. Ali, A.T. Elolemy, A.A.H. Khalil, M.K.M. Khalil, and M.S. Alqaed. 2018. "The Medical Perspective of Cupping Therapy: Effects and Mechanisms of Action," *Journal of Traditional and Complementary Medicine* 9 (2):90–97 (April). doi:10.1016/j.jtcme.2018.03.003

Fogli, A. Translation from the French. 1992. "Orbicularis Osculi Muscle and Crow's Feet: Pathogenesis and Surgical Approach," *Annales de Chirugie Plastique Esthetique* 37 (5):510–8 (Oct).

Prager, W. 2013. "Differential Characteristics of IncobotulinumtoxinA and Its Use in the Management of Glabellar Frown Lines." *Journal of Clinical Pharmacology* 5:39–52. doi: 10.2147/CPAA.S37582

RESOURCES

These suppliers carry pitcher-shaped silicone facial cups and will ship to addresses in Canada and the United States.

Carbo Medical Supplies: www.carbo.ca

Opis Supplies: www.opis-supplies.ca

Diatech: www.diatechusa.com (for Lucas-Cide sanitizer/disinfectant)

ACKNOWLEDGMENTS

I WOULD LIKE to thank Khadija, Piya, Rafique, Roger, Rosa, Sasha, Susan and Tanisha for donating all your beautiful faces to this project.

With sincere gratitude I would like to thank my mother, Jackie, my father, Tom, and Marie, my brother Jason and his wife, Paula, my darling nephews Jacob & Evan and Ethan, and dear Rafique for all of your patience and support during this process.

Thank you to all my friends who were patient and understanding during the writing process, especially Tanisha, Sista Vickie, Khadija, Sasha, Roger, Kassy and Ja(cob). And a huge thank you to my colleagues Stacie Nevelus and Lauren Lane for supporting me and our educational company while I focused on balancing the book work, classes and my private practice.

Thank you to Doug Arcos photography for capturing it all and producing such a beautiful product. And last but not least, thank you to Kathleen Fraser for editing, Kevin Cockburn for the design and Bob Dees and the rest of the Robert Rose staff for making it all possible.

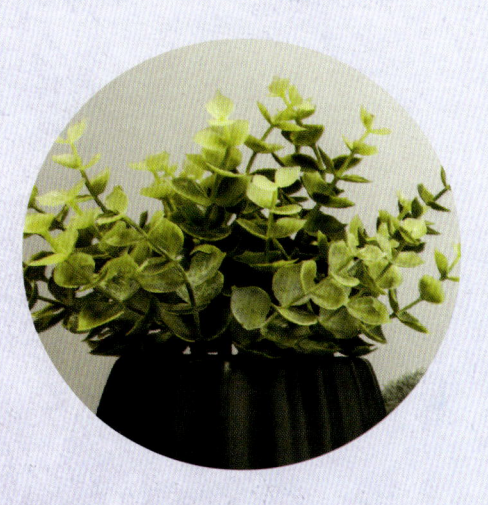

INDEX

A
acne, 79, 87
adhesions, 27
anterior triangle, 68–70

B
Bell's palsy, 87
blood vessels, 22–23
Botox. *See* cosmetic injections

C
cardiovascular system, 22–23
cheeks, 121, 126–29
chest (upper), 105–9
circulatory system, 27, 31
  cupping and, 36, 39
  facial, 22–24, 71
collagen, 20
cosmetic injections, 72, 82–83
cupping, 14. *See also* cupping techniques; cups
  benefits, 35–40, 161–62
  endangerment sites, 68–71
  marks from, 63–65
  overview, 91–93
  physiological responses to, 35–36
  preparing for, 84
  resources, 167
  results, 53, 159
  skincare after, 154–57
  step-by-step instructions, 103–50
  treatment length, 62, 65
  treatment plan, 158–59
cupping techniques, 52–62, 64–65. *See also* Universal Pass
  cup-free, 60, 77, 100–101
  lift-and-release, 53–55
  Morse Code of Cups, 59, 60
  moving/sliding, 56–58, 62, 64
cups, 44–46
  cleaning and storing, 48–49
  size of, 64, 131

D
dehydration, 30
dermatitis, 87

E

elastin, 20
endangerment sites, 68–70
exfoliation, 157
eye area
   above, 146–49
   below, 142–45
eyebrows, 78

F

face. *See also specific parts*
   anatomy of, 20–27, 71
   circulation in, 22–24, 71
   hair on, 77–78
   muscles of, 27
   skin of, 20–21
   temporal region, 71, 76
facelifts. *See* plastic surgery
fascia, 21, 27
fibroblasts, 20
forehead, 131–39

G

Gilmartin, Shannon, 17, 161–62

H

hair (facial), 77–78
hydration, 28, 30

J

jawline
   above, 116–19
   below, 112–15
jaw tension, 81

L

line of movement, 56
lip (upper), 121–25
lubricant oils, 46–47, 56, 84
lymphatic system, 23–24, 31
   cupping and, 36, 39

M

masks. *See* skincare
microcirculation, 36
moles, 76
muscles, 26–27, 95
   cupping and, 40

N

neck, 68–70, 105–9
neuralgia (trigeminal), 87
nutrition, 28, 30

O

oils, 46–47, 56, 84
   removing, 157

P

pimples, 79
plastic surgery, 73, 83, 87
posterior triangle, 69–70

R

rosacea, 87

S

scars, 161–62
sinuses, 80, 132–35
skin. *See also* skincare
  anatomy of, 20–21
  assessing, 76
  cupping and, 37
  dry, 76
  healthy, 28
  loose, 76, 82
  preparing for cupping, 84
  risks to, 30
  wrinkled, 27, 40
skincare, 28, 154–57
skin tags, 76
surgical procedures, 73, 83, 87

T

temporal region, 71, 76
throat, 68–70
TMJ dysfunction, 81
trigeminal neuralgia, 87

U

Universal Pass, 52, 56, 94–101
  cup-free option, 100–101
  rules of application, 96
  technique, 98–99

V

vasodilation, 36
veins, 22–23

W

wrinkles, 27, 40

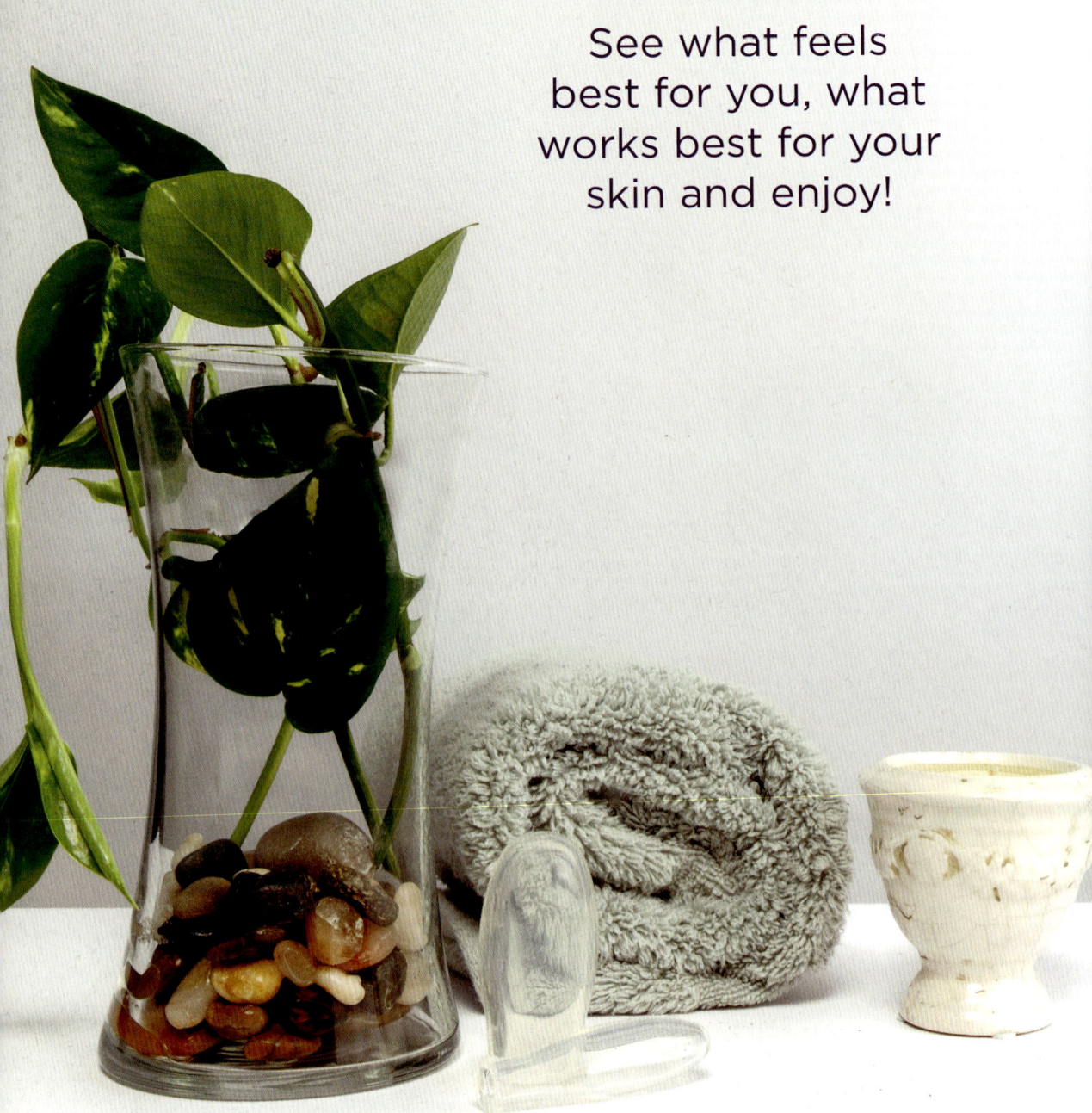

See what feels best for you, what works best for your skin and enjoy!

Library and Archives Canada Cataloguing in Publication

Title: Easy facial cupping at home : your simple guide for healthy, rejuvenated skin / Shannon Gilmartin, CMT, CMLDT, CMCTPE.
Names: Gilmartin, Shannon, author.
Description: Includes index.
Identifiers: Canadiana 20230187013 | ISBN 9780778807155 (softcover)
Subjects: LCSH: Cupping—Handbooks, manuals, etc. | LCSH: Face—Care and hygiene—Handbooks, manuals, etc. | LCSH: Skin—Care and hygiene—Handbooks, manuals, etc. | LCSH: Cupping—Popular works. | LCSH: Face—Care and hygiene—Popular works. | LCSH: Skin—Care and hygiene—Popular works. | LCSH: Beauty, Personal. | LCGFT: Handbooks and manuals.
Classification: LCC RM184 .G54 2023 | DDC 615.8/9—dc23